5/9/13
\1\1\ PT

D0100387

Early Sprouts

Early Sprouts

Cultivating
Healthy
Food Choices
in Young
Children

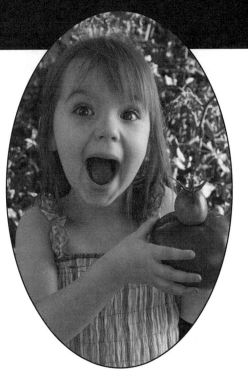

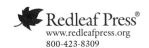 Redleaf Press®
www.redleafpress.org
800-423-8309

Published by Redleaf Press
10 Yorkton Court
St. Paul, MN 55117
www.redleafpress.org

First edition 2009
Cover design by Brad Norr Design
Interior typeset in Adobe Caslon and Geometric 415 and designed by Jim Handrigan
Illustrations by Chris Wold Dyrud and Timothy Sampson (pp. 38 and 193)

Printed in the United States of America
17 16 15 14 13 12 11 10   2 3 4 5 6 7 8 9

Library of Congress Cataloging-in-Publication Data

Kalich, Karrie.
  Early sprouts : cultivating healthy food choices in young children / Karrie Kalich, Dottie Bauer, Deirdre McPartlin.—1st ed.
       p. cm.
  Includes bibliographical references.
  ISBN 978-1-933653-72-3
  1. Preschool children—Nutrition. 2. Vegetables. 3. Food preferences. I. Bauer, Dorothy. II. McPartlin, Deirdre. III. Title.
  TX361.C5K35 2009
  649'.3—dc22
                              2008038502

Printed on acid-free paper

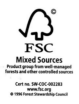

FSC
Mixed Sources
Product group from well-managed
forests and other controlled sources
Cert no. SW-COC-002283
www.fsc.org
© 1996 Forest Stewardship Council

*We dedicate this book to our own children
and the Early Sprouts children, teachers, and families.*

—Karrie, Dottie, and Deirdre

EARLY SPROUTS

Acknowledgments

Together we would like to thank all of the wonderful individuals who have contributed in such meaningful ways to the creation of this book:

The children and families at all of our Early Sprout locations.

The Keene State College Child Development Center staff: Michelle Carrio, Ellen Edge, Stacey Fortin, Karen Guiterrez, Tara Kavanagh, Carole Russell, and Carole Sands.

The many Keene State College Health Science Nutrition students who have contributed time and energy to the Early Sprouts program; Kim Foster, Jessica Lupo, and Amy Toscano, who assisted with earlier versions of the curriculum; a special thank-you to Kimberly Perry for her design of the Early Sprouts logo.

The teachers and staff of the Head Start programs in Keene, Claremont, and Drewsville, New Hampshire, and Jennifer Kozaczek and Don Hutchinson for their ongoing enthusiasm and support.

The Early Sprouts Coordinator, Lynn Arnold; and the Health Science Administrative Assistant, Sandy Sherwood.

Tracie Smith for her knowledgeable and enthusiastic gardening advice.

The generous funders who believed in and supported our work:

🌱 Advocates for Healthy Youth & Cheshire Health Foundation

🌱 CMH Foundation

🌱 Gemini Fund of the New Hampshire Charitable Foundation

🌱 Hannaford Supermarkets

- Healthy Sprouts Award from the National Gardening Association and Gardener's Supply Company
- HNH*foundation*
- Kiwanis Club of Keene, New Hampshire
- Monadnock Challenge Fund of the New Hampshire Charitable Foundation
- MacMillin, Keene, New Hampshire
- Environmental Education Fund of the New Hampshire Charitable Foundation
- National Gardening Association and Home Depot
- Stonewall Farm, Keene, New Hampshire

Suzan Schaffer Meiszner for her ongoing support, mentorship, and willingness to assist in fulfilling our Early Sprouts goals and vision.

Tim Sampson for the design and construction of so many of our Early Sprouts gardens.

Our families and close friends.

Finally, to the staff and editors at Redleaf Press for making this such a pleasurable experience.

FOREWORD

Dear Reader,

I must confess that when I first heard of the Early Sprouts program, I had my reservations. I was skeptical but at the same time hopeful. I have been an early childhood teacher for many years. Throughout those years, I have worked with children in nutrition and gardening programs with varied levels of success. The current issues of childhood obesity and the amounts of processed and highly sugared foods children consume concern me.

The Early Sprouts project is different from any other program with which I have worked. The focus on six target vegetables and the connections provided by experiencing those vegetables from seed to table have proved to be a very powerful educational experience for me and the four-year-old children with whom I work. The Early Sprouts project also has a strong connection to families and a commitment to bringing the vegetables into the home. The weekly Family Recipe Kits connect families to the curriculum in a unique way.

The commitment to the Early Sprouts program in my classroom has been comprehensive. Children have increased their consumption of the target vegetables and have grown more comfortable with unfamiliar foods. They are much more willing to taste unfamiliar foods and to talk openly and respectfully about the choices they make. We are seeing children consistently bringing butternut squash muffins, raw rainbow Swiss chard, sliced red peppers, cherry tomatoes, green beans, and carrot sticks in their lunches.

The children in my classroom have become amazing scientists as they explore the vegetables and continue to work with them throughout the year. Their abilities to observe, record data, use tools, and articulate their questions, hypotheses, and knowledge have grown incredibly. The Early Sprouts activities engage children in mathematical explorations, including counting the carrots as we harvest them, comparing the sizes of the chard leaves, and charting the characteristics of red, green, and yellow peppers. Additionally, we sing songs, write stories, draw pictures, and integrate Early Sprouts concepts throughout our classroom curriculum.

The most powerful and unexpected outcome of this curriculum has been the social relationships that have developed. Families, children, and teachers have developed a sense of community around our common experiences with the Early Sprouts activities. We look forward to exploring and cooking each week and reflect on what we know about the vegetables and the new things we are learning. Children help each other with the tools, including knives, kitchen scissors, and graters. They share thoughts on using measuring cups, filling muffin tins, and cracking eggs the best way. They are supportive and encouraging toward each other. Families ask each week about the vegetable we are working with in the classroom and look forward to the weekly Family Recipe Kit. Families also tell us that their children are participating in cooking at home and enjoying grocery shopping in the produce section of the store.

As a teacher, I have enjoyed sharing this work with children. Young children are filled with excitement about the world. They marvel at the magic of a seed sprouting, growing into a plant, flowering, and finally producing a butternut squash. As I reflected on my role as an early childhood teacher working with the Early Sprouts program, I was deeply affected by something ecologist and writer Rachel Carson wrote in her book *The Sense of Wonder* (1965): "If a child is to keep alive his inborn sense of wonder . . . he needs the companionship of at least one adult who can share it, rediscovering with him the joy, excitement, and mystery of the world we live in."

For me, the Early Sprouts program has been more than just another nutrition program. It has been a window into the learning process of young children, a new connection to their families, a scientific exploration of nature, and a fresh perspective on social relationships in the classroom and on my role as an early childhood teacher.

Sincerely,

Carole Russell
Preschool teacher

Preface

Dear Reader,

As you read this book, we invite you to learn from Carole Russell and all the other teachers, children, and families who have experienced our project, *Early Sprouts: Cultivating Healthy Food Choices in Young Children*. In the chapters that follow, we share our grand design, plant some seeds, nurture ideas, and harvest the benefits of sound nutrition, engaging early childhood curriculum, and family connections. Welcome to our journey. We're glad you can join us!

Sincerely,

Karrie, Dottie, and Deirdre
The Early Sprouts team

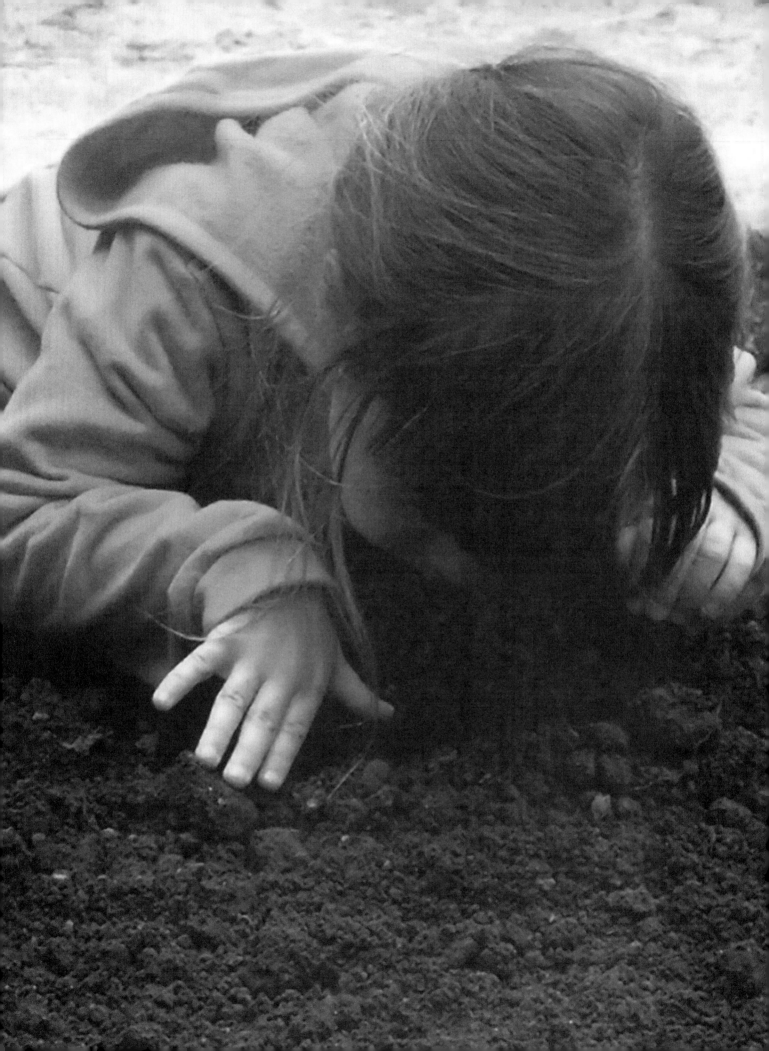

Part 1

PREPARING *the* GROUNDWORK

~ ONE ~

THE EARLY SPROUTS
PHILOSOPHY AND APPROACH

TAKE A LOOK AROUND the classroom with us. In dramatic play, Brendan and Wendy are planning a picnic. They are going to bring carrots and Swiss chard for the picnic. At the math table, Nathaniel and Cormack are working with colored pegs. "See, it's a big garden. It has carrots and tomatoes and peppers and squash and beans!" explains Cormack. Alethia is drawing in the art center. Cassie, the teacher, asks her about her drawing. Alethia replies, "This is the garden. These are the stems and roots and things you hold to eat it. I made a pumpkin too. When all the plants were picked and gone, a flower came." At the science table, Joy and Franklyn are investigating a squash plant with magnifying glasses. Joy compares the size of her hand with the size of the leaf. Franklyn comments, "The flower looks like an octopus!" At circle time, the children sing, "This is the way we plant the seeds" as they act out the planting process. Pablo and Leah share the book they've created, inspired by Eric Carle's *Today Is Monday*. Their book, called *Today Is Monday the Early Sprouts Way*, contains their drawings of garden plants. Each day has a vegetable—green beans, Swiss chard, butternut squash, tomatoes, carrots, peppers—and Sunday is for smoothies.

The *Early Sprouts: Cultivating Healthy Food Choices in Young Children* approach is based on sound nutritional research, principles of behavioral change, and a deep knowledge of early childhood curriculum. The approach involves families and provides educational opportunities for teachers and other staff who care for young children. But most important, the program is engaging and developmentally appropriate. Children's responses tell us they are interested in learning about the world

| 9

around them, gardening, preparing food, and exploring the vegetables they encounter. Teachers tell us they have learned the importance of nutrition and found the program easy to incorporate in their classrooms. And families tell us their food choices now include more vegetables. We hope you find these same successes as you try out the Early Sprouts approach.

Early Sprouts is a research-based, twenty-four-week curriculum designed to help you and your children learn about and eat vegetables. The program features organic garden beds where children plant, tend, and harvest vegetables, flowers, and herbs. We include sensory-exploration lessons featuring vegetables and healthy recipes for cooking these vegetables that were developed specifically for use with young children. Family Recipe Kits give families the opportunity to cook with their children using the same recipes—a step that builds an important home-school connection in developing healthy eating habits. Taken together, these experiences encourage children to eat more vegetables. Our classroom research demonstrates the success of the program.

Children's dietary habits are established during the early years, shaped by family preferences, lifestyle, culture, and experience. When young children spend a lot of time in group care eating snacks and meals, early childhood educators also play an important role in children's food preferences and eating habits. But how many of us intentionally try to increase children's interest in eating healthy foods, such as vegetables? How many of us implement a nutrition program that is engaging, developmentally appropriate, and tasty? How many ways can we incorporate vegetables into the learning opportunities offered in a preschool classroom or other learning environment?

Early Sprouts provides proven techniques to help classroom teachers, families, youth leaders, home child care providers, and nutritionists incorporate sensory exploration and cooking activities into the weekly curriculum. Following our curriculum will help your children and their families become familiar with the vegetables introduced in the program. Having opportunities to explore, taste, and cook these vegetables will increase children's taste preference for the vegetables you choose. By sharing the Early Sprouts approach with you, we hope to have a long-range impact on children's eating habits, resulting in a reduction in the number of overweight and obese children.

Planting the Seeds for Early Sprouts

Early Sprouts began as the brainchild of Dr. Karrie Kalich, a registered dietitian and a health science and nutrition professor at Keene State College in Keene, New Hampshire. Karrie's research on community health and her awareness of the growing obesity epidemic led to the idea of applying knowledge gained by studying the development of children's food preferences. Research indicates that it takes five to ten exposures to a new food for a young child to become comfortable with its taste and texture (Sullivan and Birch 1994). So it seemed logical that providing preschool children with multiple exposures to specific vegetables would increase their comfort with and willingness to eat these vegetables. Based on this research, Early Sprouts features six target vegetables and provides up to twelve exposures to each of the vegetables during the course of the twenty-four-week program.

In 2005, Karrie approached the Keene State College Child Development Center about the possibility of piloting a project with three important components:

1. Organic garden beds
2. A twenty-four-week curriculum of sensory explorations and cooking activities for preschoolers
3. Family Recipe Kits to help families prepare the recipes at home

In the spring of 2006, the seeds were planted, both literally and figuratively, for an ongoing partnership that has benefited all involved. As you read this book, you will find the information to help you begin the program and to establish a similar partnership:

- Guidelines for establishing garden beds
- Strategies for sensory explorations that enhance children's scientific and literacy development and provide knowledge about vegetables
- Healthy recipes specifically designed to be used with young children
- Tips for involving teachers and families in improving everyone's personal eating habits

Why Preschoolers?

Preschool children (ages two-and-a-half to five) are active learners who experience the world through their senses, physical involvement, and active play, and who learn from the behaviors modeled by adults and peers. Swiss psychologist Jean Piaget characterized children in this age range as being actively involved in constructing their knowledge of the world through hands-on experiences (Mooney 2000). They have mastered the basics of movement—walking, climbing, jumping, running—and are refining their hand-eye coordination and fine-motor skills. Preschoolers are enthusiastic about using materials, trying new experiences, and communicating their wants, needs, and ideas to others. They are able to follow directions, accomplish self-help tasks independently, and solve simple problems. At this age, they are eager to please adults, to be part of their family and community, and to make new friends (Bredekamp and Copple 1997).

Young children also have an innate food neophobia, or fear of new foods. In prehistoric times, this was a positive adaptation, because eating an unfamiliar food might result in illness or poisoning. But today, most Americans are disconnected from the source of our food supply, so we may have to intervene in order to encourage young children to try foods we know are healthy for them. By the age of five, most children have lost their innate ability to regulate the number of calories they consume and have learned to prefer foods high in fat and sugar. Advertising dollars spent on marketing sweetened cereals, soft drinks, salty snacks, and fast foods far exceed those used to promote vegetables and nutrition education programs (Gallo 1999). Children exposed to homegrown produce, however, have a higher preference for those vegetables (Nanney et al. 2007). When early childhood educators and families focus their efforts, children as well as adults can learn healthy eating habits.

Teaching Nutrition and Health

Nutrition education programs for preschoolers frequently focus on teaching children to learn the names of new foods, to classify foods using the Food Guide Pyramid (see www.mypyramid.gov), and to make healthy food choices (Marotz 2009). Government agencies, food industry groups, cooperative extension services, gardening associations, and early childhood experts promote activities, books, and Web sites that contain ideas for fun ways to introduce children to healthy foods. Some approaches involve tasting exotic foods (Bellows and Anderson 2006); others introduce different cultures through the foods eaten in them. Gardening programs provide a connection to the natural world and incorporate scientific concepts (Nimmo and Hallett 2008). Many early childhood educators also teach healthy behaviors, such as hand washing, toothbrushing, and the importance of physical activity as part of their curriculum.

National organizations responsible for excellence in early childhood education recognize the importance of nutrition and health in the preschool years. The Academy for Early Childhood Program Accreditation, sponsored by the National Association for the Education of Young Children (NAEYC), includes nutrition education as part of its Early Childhood Program Standards (Standard 2.K). (You can find more information about the NAEYC standards at www.naeyc.org/academy/standards.) Head Start expects classrooms to integrate health and nutrition into their curriculum, as stated in Regulation 1304.21 (c) (1) (iii): "Integrates all educational aspects of the health, nutrition, and mental health services into program activities." (More information on Head Start Regulations is located at http://eclkc.ohs.acf.hhs.gov/hslc.)

The Early Sprouts curriculum will help you meet these national standards. The program offers a framework of developmentally appropriate opportunities for

> **NAEYC STANDARD 2.K: CURRICULUM CONTENT AREA FOR COGNITIVE DEVELOPMENT: HEALTH AND SAFETY**
>
> 2.K.01 Children are provided varied opportunities and materials that encourage good health practices such as serving and feeding themselves, rest, good nutrition, exercise, hand washing, and tooth brushing.
>
> 2.K.02 Children are provided varied opportunities and materials to help them learn about nutrition, including identifying sources of food and recognizing, preparing, eating, and valuing healthy foods. (NAEYC 2007)

preschoolers to learn about six vegetables, referred to as *target vegetables*. The lessons are designed to engage children's senses and curiosity and to reintroduce the six vegetables throughout a twenty-four-week period. The approach has specific components; however, it also provides an open-ended opportunity for the observant teacher to build on the interests and questions of the children. In addition, Early Sprouts provides information for families and involves them in exploring the vegetables, the garden, and in preparing healthy recipes.

Teachers who value an emergent curriculum (Jones and Nimmo 1994) or the project approach (Cadwell 1997, Katz and Chard 2000) find that incorporating Early Sprouts into their classroom stimulates children's thinking and provides many new ideas for projects. Children's questions about plant growth, taste sensations, and cooking processes lead to deeper knowledge of science, math, and the natural world. Children's creative exploration leads to artwork, dramatization, stories, and songs that express their ideas about the vegetables. Cassie, the pre-K teacher whose classroom is described at the beginning of this chapter, says, "From the perspective of an early childhood teacher, this program is very holistic. It's not isolated to the Early Sprouts table. It allows us to do everything."

Seed-to-Table Approach

Early Sprouts offers a "seed-to-table" approach to nutrition education for young children. We begin in the early spring by planning the garden and replenishing the soil. Children assist in determining where to plant each vegetable and often add herbs and flowers to the garden layout. They sprout seeds, visit businesses supplying

garden products, shop for seedlings at farmers' markets and local nurseries, and plant according to a schedule appropriate for their United States Department of Agriculture (USDA) Plant Hardiness Zone. In our region, that means waiting until mid to late May to plant most seedlings. You can find information about plant hardiness zones at www.usna. usda.gov/Hardzone/.

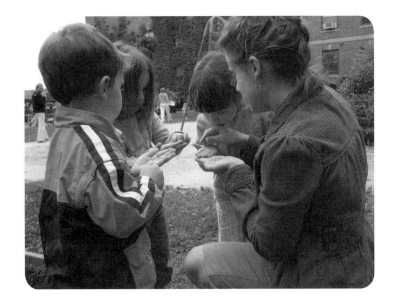

Planting seeds helps set the stage for children to understand the source of the foods they eat. As our society has become busier and less involved in food production and preparation, common knowledge of plants as food sources has diminished. Young children and their families are often more familiar with the appearance of frozen or canned vegetables than they are with fresh produce. Even many of the fresh vegetables in the produce section are wrapped in plastic or are precut for ease of use. These store-bought vegetables in all their forms—fresh, frozen, canned—often bear little resemblance to their garden relatives.

By beginning with seeds and seedlings, Early Sprouts provides a connection to the natural world that is missing in many children's lives (Louv 2005). As children participate in planting their garden, they establish a personal connection with the vegetables they are growing.

One late September day, the children in our program went out to the play yard and discovered that the carrots had been harvested in preparation for a cooking project. Darrell was so upset that he tried to plant squash leaves in the empty bed and recruited several others to help him replant the garden. (We learned our lesson and will never again harvest the vegetables without the children's involvement.)

The vegetables chosen as the six target vegetables to include in our Early Sprouts gardens have different colors and include different edible parts of plants:

VEGETABLE	COLOR(S)	PLANT PARTS
Carrots	orange	root
Swiss chard	green	leaf
	yellow, red, pink, white	stem
Green beans	green, purple, yellow	seeds and seedpod
Tomatoes	red, orange, yellow	fruit
Butternut squash	orange	fruit
Bell peppers	green, red, yellow, orange, purple	fruit

You can find additional age-appropriate information about plant parts at "My Dad's Vegetable Garden," a Web site by the Department of Biology at James Madison University at www.jmu.edu/biology/k12/garden/parts.html.

The six vegetables we've chosen to focus on grow easily in our area (USDA Hardiness Zone 5a) as well as in most other regions and are affordable and available from local growers and grocers throughout the year. By selecting readily available vegetables for the Early Sprouts curriculum, we are supporting local agriculture, being mindful of food costs, and focusing on ordinary and familiar rather than exotic foods. By selecting vegetables that grow easily, we accept the real-life gardening problems that may occur. Plants may be damaged by overenthusiastic weeding or watering or by unusual weather conditions. Garden pests such as birds, insects, or animals occasionally invade and demolish a variety of plants. Children sometimes harvest vegetables before they are ripe. In one of our Early Sprouts gardens, many of the vegetables disappeared over a weekend in late summer. We assume they were picked by a neighborhood resident. But we could still implement the curriculum because the vegetables were affordable and available.

Young children often need immediate feedback and reinforcement to learn concepts. They also need to repeat experiences to fully master them, as evidenced by the child who completes the same puzzle over and over again, each time exclaiming, "I did it!" Long-term involvement with the Early Sprouts garden provides children with direct experience and feedback over time. This regular exposure is beneficial because children have varying interests and attention spans. Planting the garden in an outdoor play area or other location close to the classroom offers easy and frequent contact with the growing plants. Visiting the garden on a regular basis allows teachers to respond to children's interests rather than require that everyone participate on a specific day. Visits also provide the repetition that strengthens young children's learning. Teachers report that each time they revisit a vegetable, the children's explorations and questions go deeper.

Caring for the garden leads to math and science lessons about plant growth and the natural world. It provides the opportunity to observe the changes to the stems, leaves, flowers, and fruits of the various vegetables over several months' time. Four-year-old Judd dragged his favorite teacher over to the garden beds. "Liza, you gotta come see this." They stopped by the squash vine, and he moved a leaf to reveal a large tan butternut squash. "What is it?" asked Liza. "I don't know, but you gotta look at it!" was his reply.

Measuring the plants and recording their growth with graphs, photographs, and drawings provides documentation of the process for children, families, and caregivers. Weeding and cultivating the soil support classifying plants into edible and nonedible categories and give children responsibility for the care of the garden. Identifying insects, birds, butterflies, small mammals, and other creatures visiting the garden expands children's knowledge of living things and builds observation skills and a connection to nature. Robyn wondered about the holes she saw in a Swiss chard leaf and observed, "Maybe a caterpillar chewed it. Do caterpillars like chard?"

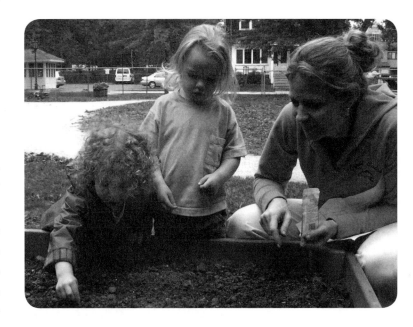

Harvesting the ripe vegetables celebrates the growing season and the children's efforts. Children are involved in picking individual vegetables and in pulling out the plants at the end of the growing season. Doing the real work of harvesting supports the development of a positive self-concept and an understanding of the importance of working together. At the end of the growing season, it takes four or five children all pulling together to get the squash and tomato vines out of the ground. Composting the remains of the plants and the inedible parts of each vegetable brings knowledge of decomposition and nourishment of the soil. This connects the children to the natural cycles of life and death and to the concepts of weather and the four seasons. The harvest creates a transition between sensory exploration of the garden and cooking components of the Early Sprouts curriculum, leading us from the seed to the table.

As a new school year begins in the autumn, we begin the structured part of the curriculum with the garden's mature plants. Some children may have participated in planting them the previous spring or in maintaining them with their families during the summer. Other children may not have had any experience with the garden. Waiting for a garden to grow and produce fruit takes a long time. We believe children need a more immediate introduction to vegetables at the beginning of the program, so we suggest starting with full-grown vegetables.

Of course, you can reap the benefits of the Early Sprouts program even without starting an actual garden. (Chapter 3 provides ideas for small-scale outdoor and indoor growing, while chapter 14 offers suggestions for making Early Sprouts work in a variety of settings.)

Sensory Exploration

Young children learn through their senses and through movement. Actively involving the children in sensory exploration of vegetables is an important component of the Early Sprouts curriculum. By sensory exploration we mean intentionally and actively using all of our senses to interact with and experience a food. In this way, Early Sprouts contributes to young children's brain growth and development. Sensation, or the intake of information through the senses, provides the input needed for learning and understanding. Perception is the way in which the brain makes sense of the input it receives. Sensory explorations and cooking activities

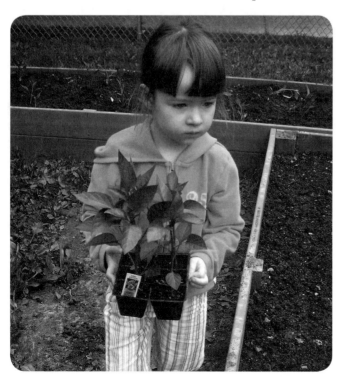

provide multiple sensations, which in turn lead to perceptions. This process leads to the growth of neuronal connections in the brain, making way for thinking, processing, memory, problem solving, and other important brain functions. The early years are the most important times for brain development, and Early Sprouts provides very important sensory stimulation necessary to healthy development during this period.

Besides stimulating the traditional five senses—sight, hearing, touch, smell, taste—Early Sprouts also stimulates children's perceptions of temperature, body awareness, and kinesthetic sense, known as *proprioception*, into the program. Each of these senses contributes its share to the child's knowledge of the vegetables. Early Sprouts provides many opportunities for children to develop their senses, stimulate their brains, and integrate their various senses through sensory explorations, cooking, and tasting.

Sensory explorations in the Early Sprouts program focus on each vegetable as a vegetable. Questions are posed, such as "What is inside?" and children are encouraged to make predictions, an activity that stimulates scientific thinking. Teachers promote language development by using descriptive words—*crunchy, crisp, smooth, sweet, slippery*—to explain what the children are seeing, touching, hearing, tasting, and smelling.

One group of children decided to count all the seeds inside the bell peppers they were exploring. They became interested in the differences in shape and color of those seeds. This simple activity—cutting open bell peppers—engaged the children for more than half an hour.

Charts and graphs of plant growth or taste testing foster mathematical thinking. Organizing the various shapes and sizes of carrots—short, long, fat, thin, single, double—becomes a lesson in classification by size, shape, and color. We examine the vegetables in different forms—cooked, raw, dried, fresh, grated, sliced—and compare and contrast the plant parts, the cooking techniques, and the tastes, colors, smells, and textures we experience. Zuri noted, "The raw chard has a little juice. The cooked chard is softer and easy to break." And Maisy commented, "They both taste different. The raw tastes drier and the cooked tastes sweeter."

We want to emphasize that we do not use vegetables as play objects in the Early Sprouts program. Some early childhood classrooms incorporate food items into the art curriculum, such as printing with vegetables and fruits or creating collages with pasta shapes. In addition to sand and water, their sensory tables may feature grains or seeds such as cornmeal, rice, and birdseed for children's tactile stimulation. Some early childhood educators and programs do not use food as a curriculum material. Sometimes this decision is based on philosophical grounds—children are hungry, and food should be used for nourishment only. Other times it results from an analysis of cognitive development—young children can't distinguish between food to eat and food to play with, so they risk biting a potato with paint on it or eating the rice at the sensory table.

In the Early Sprouts curriculum, we do not play with vegetables. Instead, we explore and investigate them. Our approach to sensory exploration is for children to use their senses, with intentional guidance from caring adults, to directly understand and experience a particular vegetable in all its forms as a vegetable, not as an art material or an implement. By focusing on the vegetable's characteristics and qualities, we believe we are adding to children's knowledge and understanding of vegetables as foods. This relates to one of our main goals, which is to provide young children with multiple exposures to each vegetable to increase their preference for and willingness to eat it.

Cooking and Recipe Development

The recipes used each week in the Early Sprouts program were specifically developed to reflect healthy nutritional principles and contain affordable ingredients. They were also designed for cooking with young children and feature simple directions that maximize the children's ability to participate in making the recipe. The recipes are easy to prepare, so families can cook with their child using the Family Recipe Kits.

Each recipe features one of the six target vegetables used in our curriculum. In addition, the recipes include these healthful ingredients:

- Whole grains, such as stone-ground cornmeal, brown rice, whole grain pasta, and whole wheat flour
- Reduced amounts of sodium and sugars compared to those in commercially prepared snack foods
- Low-fat dairy products, such as skim milk or low-fat plain yogurt
- Oils containing healthy fats, such as canola, safflower, or olive

These ingredient choices are based on the Food Guide Pyramid (www.mypyramid.gov) and recommendations from the American Dietetic Association (www.eatright.org).

We also emphasize healthy food preparation techniques. Vegetables are steamed rather than boiled, for example, and quesadillas are baked or broiled rather than fried. The recipes were field-tested with preschool children and teachers prior to being adopted as part of the program. In addition, they are revised each year, based on feedback about how the recipes taste, how easy they are to follow for a group of children, and how much time is required to prepare them. We welcome your ideas for improvements on the recipes as well. (Our contact information is included on page 203.)

Recipes vary in preparation time, the tools used, the number of steps required, and the variety of ingredients included. Vegetables served with a special dip or incorporated into smoothies are relatively easy to prepare in the classroom; muffins and pasta dishes take longer. All of the recipes are designed to be used as a snack or part of a lunch meal. Recipes yield eighteen child-sized servings. The curriculum begins with simple recipes—for example, Cherry Tomatoes with Honey Mustard Dip—and progresses to more complex, multistep cooking projects, such as Carrot Oatmeal Cookies. Some recipes have creative names designed to motivate children's participation, such as Bell Pepper Couscous Castles. Other names describe the ingredients or recognizable prepared foods, such as Cheddar and Chard Quesadillas or Green Bean Wontons with Dipping Sauce.

We find that children are very capable of doing the real work of food preparation, if the adults responsible for their care and education take a little time to plan for their participation. The cooking tools we use are selected with safety and success in mind. Children use table knives with fine serrations and stir with long-handled wooden spoons. They use graters to shred carrots or cheese and child-sized kitchen scissors to cut greens. They operate the blender or food processor only with adult supervision. Each recipe for cooking with children includes tips that have been field tested by experienced preschool teachers.

Sanitation is very important in the Early Sprouts program. We emphasize the importance of hand washing before handling food, after tasting, after sneezing or coughing on hands, and after touching something that might be dirty, such as shoes or something that fell on the floor. We do not use any raw meat products in our recipes, so the issue of cross-contamination or infection from undercooked meats does not come up. Research indicates that young children usually don't know when they need to wash their hands; however, when they are taught the importance of proper hand washing, they are eager to comply (Witt and Spencer 2004). For that reason, it is important to teach about hand washing and remind children to wash their hands whenever they participate in an Early Sprouts activity.

> **HOW TO WASH YOUR HANDS**
>
> 1. Wet your hands with warm running water.
> 2. Apply soap.
> 3. Wash your hands for at least twenty seconds. Sing the entire "ABC Song" while you rub the fronts and backs of your hands and your fingers, thumbs, and wrists.
> 4. Rinse your hands with the fingertips pointing down so the soap goes down the drain.
> 5. Turn the faucet off with a paper towel so you don't get your hands dirty again.
> 6. Dry your hands with a clean paper towel.
> 7. Throw the paper towel in the trash.

Family Involvement

The Early Sprouts program recognizes that families play a significant role in the development of young children's food likes and dislikes (Birch and Fisher 1996). Families are vitally important in the care and education of young children. They provide an intergenerational, inclusive environment in which children interact and learn from people of all ages and abilities in the home. Families are the child's first and most important teachers and, as such, they provide the context for early feeding and food choices. They model eating habits every time they select, prepare, and eat meals, shaping children's future eating habits. If as early childhood educators we want to have a positive impact on the children we teach, we must find positive ways to connect with their families.

We recognize that families with young children face many challenges to developing healthful eating habits, including limited time and knowledge to prepare nutritious meals. They are bombarded by fast-food and food-product suppliers' marketing, and they may not know how to influence picky eaters. Through the Early Sprouts program, we share knowledge with families. (Chapter 5 describes the accepting approach we use to discuss these issues and educate families. It also details the communication, events, and feedback opportunities the program includes to encourage family participation.)

As part of Early Sprouts, children help pack a Family Recipe Kit to take home. Four-year-old Andrea, who really likes to cook, asks regularly, "Are we taking home ingredients today?" The recipe kit contains key ingredients, along with detailed instructions for preparing the recipe at home. Families are encouraged to cook with their child to reinforce the classroom experience. The kit provides families with healthful recipes along with guidance and support for cooking with their preschoolers. Cooking at home also provides opportunities for the child to taste the food again and to connect the school activity to the family table. Three-year-old Martin was crushed one evening, according to his mother, when she served couscous to the family. "But Mom, there aren't peppers in it," he sobbed. "Couscous castles have peppers." (You will find the recipes for and further information about Family Recipe Kits in chapter 12.)

Families are informed of the Early Sprouts activities through monthly newsletter articles. They can participate in garden planting, classroom-based sensory and cooking activities, family nutrition education programming, and food-based special events, such as a stone soup luncheon. At the end of the year, families receive a cookbook containing all of the Early Sprouts weekly recipes. (You will also find details about these opportunities for family participation in chapter 5.)

What Our Research Tells Us

Early Sprouts provides educational and motivational activities for preschool children to help them learn about vegetables, gardening, and cooking. Our research protocol has demonstrated that the curriculum increases children's willingness to try vegetables. The results also indicate an increase in children's preference for the six target vegetables we have used. Although you certainly don't need to include

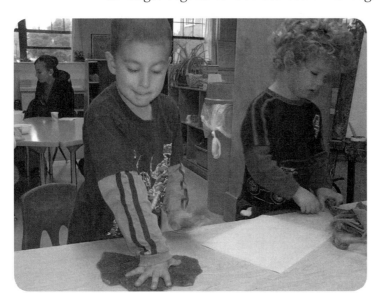

the research aspect of the program when you implement the curriculum, we want to explain how that work has been accomplished. The research results may encourage families to make personal changes and motivate program administrators and policy makers to support the program.

As part of testing the Early Sprouts model, we conducted food-preference assessments of children three times each year. The entire program provides between eight and twelve exposures to each target vegetable. Our results indicate that children's willingness to try the vegetables increases and so does their positive reaction to each vegetable. While some vegetables—for example, carrots and beans—are more familiar at the outset, children's preference for all six target vegetables showed a significant increase at the program's conclusion.

Other aspects of the research involve gathering feedback from families and classroom teachers. (Chapter 5 includes examples of our feedback forms, and chapter 13 contains a more detailed explanation of the research and a summary of our results.)

Now that you have an overview of the Early Sprouts philosophy and approach, you are ready to learn more about the nutrition concepts that inspired the creation of the program. The next chapter explores the motivation behind Early Sprouts and reviews basic nutritional guidelines for young children.

TWO

THE NUTRITIONAL APPROACH

ONVINCING CHILDREN to eat the right foods is often challenging. Surprisingly, well-intentioned adults often contribute to children's poor dietary choices, both in terms of the quantity and quality of foods eaten, by using food as a bribe or reward. Coercive approaches may work in the short-term—the child may eat the vegetables on a given night. But in the long run, adults have not helped the child learn to consume these foods by choice and to establish eating vegetables as a part of daily life.

Instilling healthy eating behaviors in preschool children through a positive approach assists them in the development of lifelong habits. These healthy habits will decrease their risk of obesity and other chronic diseases. To encourage such positive lifelong habits, the Early Sprouts program builds on the following nutritional background and public health practices.

The Obesity Epidemic

The increase in the percentage of the United States population that is either overweight or obese is one of the fastest growing public health concerns. Early childhood educators have not usually considered children's weight to be significant in their work and have often been warned not to emphasize issues of weight in the preschool years. But that is changing. In fact, medical and public health professionals are more and more concerned about the rise in childhood obesity. Some of the most dramatic increases in the number of overweight and obese Americans are found among preschool-aged children, whose obesity has more than doubled in the past thirty years (Penn State Live 2005). This problem is reaching epidemic proportions.

Obesity in children and adults has many causes. The major factors contributing to childhood obesity fall into two broad categories: 1) too little physical activity and 2) poor dietary habits. Children are too sedentary and consuming too many sugared and processed foods that are high in calories and low in nutritional value. Although Early Sprouts encourages outdoor physical activity by involving young children in the physical work associated with planting, maintaining, and harvesting a garden, the primary focus of our project is promoting healthy dietary habits. These include increasing the consumption of vegetables, fruits, low-fat dairy products, healthy fats, and whole grains. Early Sprouts uses multiple approaches to promote, encourage, and support healthier food choices that ultimately result in a healthy body weight and a reduced risk of chronic illnesses, such as diabetes and heart disease.

The Importance of Starting Early

Some people question our focus on preschool children, suggesting that we should direct our efforts toward older children, who are better able to understand the importance of a healthy diet. Although understanding the value of healthy eating is important, it is even more important that children (and adults) actually make good dietary choices. Many people with sufficient knowledge about healthy foods are unable to succeed in consistently following a healthy diet. Older children typically must first overcome already established poor eating habits and then work to establish new, healthier habits. As a nation, we need strategies that support people to take their knowledge and put it into action, to help them change their behaviors with regard to food preferences and patterns.

In many ways, the preschool years constitute the ideal time to inspire the development of healthy eating habits. During this developmental period, young children first establish many of the eating habits they will practice for the rest of their lives. When children are provided with healthy food choices and allowed to determine how much they consume (without external pressure to eat or not eat), they are able to self-regulate how many calories they consume (Johnson and Birch 1994). Simply put, a very young child will suddenly stop eating a favorite food because he is full. As children become increasingly aware of the world around them and as external messages around food become more evident, their ability to self-regulate decreases. Preschool children become more likely to want a food because a friend or family member is eating it or because they have seen it advertised. They learn to eat because it is mealtime and are less likely to respond to their own internal cues about being hungry or satiated. This makes the preschool years an appropriate time to teach healthy eating through modeling healthy behaviors and offering opportunities to try healthy foods. It is much easier and more effective to teach healthy dietary behaviors than to work to change unhealthy ones.

Healthy Eating for Preschool Children

The United States Department of Agriculture (USDA), creator of the USDA Food Guide Pyramid, publishes guidelines for a healthy diet on its Web site, www.mypyramid.gov. The recently revised 2005 Food Guide Pyramid illustrates the relative importance of different foods within a healthy diet and reflects current research on the importance of various nutrients and foods. The Web site allows you to customize dietary recommendations, plan menus, and find nutritional resources. The pyramid recommends that daily intake should include elements from these five food groups:

- Grains, half of which should be whole grains
- Vegetables
- Fruits
- Dairy products
- Protein-rich foods, such as lean meats, poultry, and fish, and dry beans, legumes, and nuts

Varying the types of these foods on a weekly basis contributes to a healthy diet. For example, dark green leafy vegetables and orange vegetables supply different important nutrients. Both are not needed each day, but both should be included in weekly menus. Fresh fruits are preferred, and fruit juices should be limited because of their extra sugar content. It is also important to limit extras, such as sugary foods and snacks, and to include healthy oils while decreasing consumption of trans and saturated fats. The USDA recommends exercise as an important component of the healthy diet.

The USDA makes different dietary recommendations based on age, activity level, and gender. Adults need to remember that children have different dietary needs from their own, both in portion size and nutritional composition. For example, preschool children should consume three servings of vegetables and two servings of fruit daily. The Food Guide Pyramid recommends that young children consume two each day of

---

DEFINITIONS OF *VEGETABLE* AND *FRUIT*

According to botanists, the part of a plant that bears the seed is considered the *fruit*. In the terms of plant science, this means that several of our target vegetables are actually fruits. Tomatoes, green beans, butternut squash, and bell peppers all grow from the fertilized flower of the plant, and they produce and contain the seeds for the next generation of that plant.

Botanists do not define the term *vegetable*. According to various dictionaries, *vegetables* are the edible parts of plants, and *fruits* are the parts of flowering plants containing the seeds. Nutritionists, grocery stores, cookbooks, and parents use both words to mean the edible parts of some plants we should eat daily. We usually distinguish vegetables from fruits by describing fruits as sweet and fleshy, while vegetables are characterized as more bitter and savory in flavor.

All of our target vegetables can be described as vegetables—the edible parts of plants. Swiss chard is the stem and leaf of the plant, while carrots are the roots. The rest are technically fruits.

It's not surprising that this distinction is confusing. The U.S. Supreme Court actually heard a case in the nineteenth century in which the tomato was defined as a vegetable. The case involved tariffs levied on imported vegetables but not on imported fruits (*Nix v. Hedden*, 149 U.S. 304, 1893). If the tomato was a fruit, it was exempt from the tariff; if it was a vegetable, the importers owed the tax.

All of this means we are using different meanings of the word *fruit* when we talk about eating fruit, experiencing the fruits of our labors, or harvesting the fruits of the vegetable plants. Each meaning is correct, as long as we keep its context in mind.

low-fat or fat-free dairy products. It also recommends that young children consume six daily servings of bread, rice, or pasta, half of these whole grains. The following chart summarizes the Food Guide Pyramid recommendations for a typical four-year-old child.

SERVING AMOUNTS AND SIZES RECOMMENDED BY THE USDA FOOD GUIDE PYRAMID FOR AN AVERAGE FOUR-YEAR-OLD BASED ON A 1,400-CALORIE DIET (www.mypyramid.gov/mypyramid/index.aspx)

FOOD GROUP	DAILY AMOUNT	FOOD ITEM SUGGESTIONS
Grain group	5 ounces	bread ready-to-eat cereal cooked cereal, rice, or pasta
Vegetable group	1.5 cups	raw leafy vegetables other vegetables, cooked or raw vegetable juice
Fruit group	1.5 cups	medium apple, banana, orange, or pear chopped, cooked, or canned fruit fruit juice
Milk group (preferably fat-free or low-fat)	2 cups	2 cups milk or yogurt natural cheese, such as cheddar processed cheese, such as American
Meat and Beans group (preferably fat-free or low-fat)	4 ounces	lean meat, poultry, or fish The following count as 1 ounce of meat: ½ cup of cooked dry beans or tofu 2½-ounce soy burger 1 egg 2 tablespoons of peanut butter 1/3 cup of nuts

Dietitians and public health officials recommend a diet rich in fruits and vegetables partly because these foods help people achieve and maintain healthy body weights. Fresh fruits and vegetables provide vitamins, minerals, and fiber without contributing too many calories to one's total daily intake. These nutrient-dense foods are important in young children's diets because of their high vitamin and mineral content, which supports healthy physical growth and development. (*Nutrient-dense* means that a serving provides a significant amount of important nutrients compared to the number of calories provided.) Total calories and activity level are also related. When a person eats more calories than are used in activities of daily living and daily exercise, he or she gains weight. When fewer calories are eaten than used, the person loses weight.

The Early Sprouts curriculum has chosen to focus on vegetables because of their importance in healthy eating. Vegetables are naturally somewhat bitter in flavor, whereas fruits taste sweeter because of their fruit sugar or fructose. Young children prefer eating fruit to vegetables. The preference some children show for vegetables is among the strongest predictors of vegetable consumption (Birch 1979, Morris and Zidenberg-Cherr 2002). This research suggested the core component of the Early Sprouts program: to increase vegetable consumption, we must support children in preferring vegetables instead of high-fat and sugary snack foods.

Fruits and vegetables are important to eat because they are natural sources of essential vitamins, minerals, and fiber. In fact, consuming a diet rich in fruits and vegetables helps to protect us against several chronic diseases. Compared to people who consume a minimal amount of fruits and vegetables, those who eat generous amounts have decreased risk of cardiovascular diseases, strokes, and certain cancers. (Chapter 6 contains the specific nutrient information for each of the six target vegetables in the Early Sprouts curriculum.) Appendix A, page 189, contains a chart of vitamins and selected minerals and their health benefits.

VEGETABLES

To maximize the nutritional benefit of vegetables, a wide variety should be consumed. Vegetables of different colors provide different nutrients. Orange carrots and butternut squash are rich sources of beta carotene. Red tomatoes are an excellent source of vitamin C. Green Swiss chard is a good source of iron and potassium. All vegetables are a good source of dietary fiber. Canned vegetables lose some of their vitamin content during processing and tend to be high in sodium. Canned vegetables without added salt can be a part of a healthy diet. Overall, fresh, frozen, or unsalted canned vegetables are recommended.

FRUIT

It is also important to eat a wide variety of fruit. Eating different colors and types each day contributes to a healthy diet because different fruits provide

---

The 2005 *Dietary Guidelines for Americans* recommend that less than 1 teaspoon, or 2,300 milligrams, of sodium be consumed per day. Here are some tips for limiting sodium:

- Choose fresh or frozen fruits and vegetables, or canned fruits and vegetables with no added salt

- Select unsalted nuts and nut butters

- Add minimal amounts of salt when cooking; instead, season with fresh or dried herbs and spices

- Cook rice, pasta, and hot cereals without salt

- Rinse canned foods to remove some of the sodium

- Choose a ready-to-eat breakfast cereal that is lower in sodium

- Cook with whole foods; minimize the amount of processed and packaged foods consumed

- Reduce the amount of salt in all recipes by at least half; if a recipe contains baking soda or powder, eliminate all of the salt

- Use products made without added sodium

- Snack on fresh fruits and vegetables instead of salty chips and crackers

- Select low-sodium cheeses

- Remove the salt shaker from the kitchen table

Note: It takes our taste buds a few weeks to adjust to a low-sodium diet. After two to three weeks of a reduced sodium diet, most people wonder how they ever consumed such salty foods.

different nutrients. For example, bananas are a rich source of potassium; citrus fruits are an excellent source of vitamin C. Choosing whole or cut-up fruit is more nutritious than drinking fruit juice. Whole fruits are richer in dietary fiber and lower in total sugar per serving than juice. When possible, chose fresh or frozen (without added sugar) fruit instead of canned fruit. Canned fruit without added sugar and packed in its own juice, however, can also contribute to a healthy diet.

WHOLE GRAINS

In addition to fruits and vegetables, whole grains are important for maintaining health. Whole grains include barley, bulgur, brown rice, cornmeal, millet, oatmeal, spelt, white whole-wheat flour, whole-grain cereals, whole-grain pasta, whole-wheat couscous, and whole-wheat flour (red wheat). As preschoolers, children can learn to enjoy whole grains. These habits and taste preferences will help them sustain healthy eating patterns as they mature and become adults themselves.

Whole grains contain more vitamins, minerals, and dietary fiber than processed grains, such as bleached or unbleached all-purpose flour, white rice, and durum semolina pasta. They are a more complete source of nutrition than their processed cousins. Processed grains have the bran and germ removed by polishing. These nutritional components are then sold separately, in forms such as wheat germ or bran cereal. An easy way to add whole grains to your diet is to substitute them for processed grains you are already eating.

Many health benefits are associated with consuming dietary fiber from fruits, vegetables, and whole grains. For example, take dietary fiber:

> ᘯ Improves bowel function
>
> ᘯ Reduces the risk of developing hemorrhoids and diverticula (small pouches on the inside of the colon)
>
> ᘯ Contributes to the maintenance of a healthy weight
>
> ᘯ Reduces the risk of obesity by making us feel full without a lot of calories
>
> ᘯ Assists with regulating blood sugar levels
>
> ᘯ Helps manage blood cholesterol levels
>
> ᘯ Reduces the risk of colon cancer

SUBSTITUTING WHOLE GRAINS FOR PROCESSED GRAINS

- Use brown rice, spelt, or wheat berries instead of white rice

- Choose a whole-grain cereal, such as oatmeal, instead of a processed-grain cereal

- Select stone-ground whole-wheat bread instead of white bread

- Replace one-third to one-half of the all-purpose flour in your favorite recipes with white whole-wheat or whole-wheat flour

- Exchange 100 percent of the all-purpose flour in a favorite recipe with whole-wheat pastry flour

- Substitute whole-grain pastas for white pastas

- Use barley instead of noodles in soups

Look for dietary fiber on food labels. Try to choose products with 2 to 5 grams of fiber per serving.

DAIRY

Low-fat dairy products are important for maintaining health. Preschoolers can learn to enjoy 1- or 2-percent or fat-free dairy products, such as milk or yogurt, to establish this healthy habit and taste preference early.

Dairy-based foods are a rich source of calcium and vitamin D. Both of these nutrients are important for bone growth and development. Calcium is also important for blood clotting, transmission of nerve impulses, and muscle contraction. It may play a role in maintaining a healthy weight. Many dairy products, such as whole milk, whole-milk yogurt, cream, half-and-half, sour cream, cream cheese, and ice cream, are also sources of saturated fat. This type of fat is a key contributor to heart disease. For that reason, low-fat or fat-free calcium-rich foods are a key component of a healthy diet. Since every cell in our body needs calcium, it is important to consume low-fat or nonfat dairy products on a daily basis. Fat-free and low-fat milk, cheeses, and yogurts are good choices.

For those who are lactose intolerant or have a dairy allergy, many dairy-free alternatives are available. Select fortified soy or rice products. The quality and variety of these products are constantly improving. Be sure to select a product that is fortified with calcium and vitamin D but not loaded with added sugars.

When buying flavored yogurt, be mindful of the sugar content. Many of the fruited yogurts currently available contain more than 3 tablespoons of sugar per serving. The USDA recommends that we consume sugar in moderation because sugar contains empty calories, meaning it is high in calories but low in vitamins and minerals. If you find eating plain yogurt less enjoyable, add fresh fruit to it or combine plain yogurt with some of your favorite fruited yogurt.

> Remember that 12 grams of sugar = 1 tablespoon.

Vitamin D, the sunshine vitamin, is as important as calcium for bone growth and development. In fact, without vitamin D calcium cannot be absorbed by our bones. Exposing hands, arms, and face to the sun provides vitamin D. In northern climates during the winter months, a negligible amount of vitamin D is available from sunlight, so it must be consumed through food. Common food items including fat-free or low-fat milk and milk products, fortified breakfast cereals, and eggs can help us meet our vitamin D needs.

Sadly, children's diets are typically high in saturated fat, sodium, and added sugars, and low in fruits, vegetables, and whole grains (Enns, Mickle, and Goldman 2002). On average, preschool children consume approximately two servings of vegetables and only one and a half servings of fruit each day. Compare this to the recommendation that preschoolers eat three to five servings of vegetables and two to four servings of fruit daily. Only 1 percent of preschool children meet all of the dietary recommendations established by the Food Guide Pyramid (Muñoz et al. 1997). This dismal statistic indicates that much needs to be done to improve young children's diets. Early Sprouts has been designed to incorporate healthy nutritional principles and practices to help address this problem.

The Early Sprouts Nutritional Philosophy

To help young children and their families establish healthy dietary behaviors, we based the Early Sprouts program on an understanding of how young children establish their food preferences. Three major factors contribute to the dietary habits of young children:

1. The innate presence of food neophobia (fear of new foods)
2. The increased influence of environmental and social messages about food
3. The approaches used by many well-intentioned adults when offering foods to young children

We have designed our program to take these factors into account and to provide strategies that help shift young children's food preferences in a positive, healthy direction. We address food neophobia, suggest positive ways to use healthy environmental and social influences on preschoolers, and provide alternative techniques for adults trying to encourage children's healthy eating.

Neophobia, the fear of new things, has evolutionary roots stemming back to the Paleolithic era of hunting and gathering. When it came to food supply, early humans did not necessarily know whether newly encountered foods would be nourishing or poisonous. Those who were cautious when encountering a new food source were more likely to survive; those who tried everything might become ill or die from ingesting a poisonous, contaminated, or rotten food. Even in the face of starvation, survival-oriented humans were not too eager to consume what could be a lethal food. As a result, our Paleolithic ancestors developed fear of unknown foods, or food neophobia, and this became part of our genetic makeup.

Children still experience an exaggerated level of food neophobia. Food neophobia is especially present when children are exposed to bitter-tasting foods. In times before modern scientific knowledge, if the fruit from a plant tasted sweet, it was considered probably safe to eat; if it tasted sour or bitter, it was better to proceed with great caution. Many vegetables have a slightly bitter flavor, whereas fruits tend to taste sweeter. Therefore, young children are naturally more accepting of fruits than vegetables—and even more naturally accepting of cookies, candy, soda, ice cream, and other sweetened foods. Most often, children who are not eating sufficient amounts of fruit are doing so because fruit is not being offered. The "bitterness" of vegetables requires a slightly different and more strategic approach. Repeated, nonthreatening opportunities to taste a new food or vegetable provide the opportunity and possibility for children to alter their reactions from rejection to acceptance (Birch and Marlin 1982, Sullivan and Birch 1994).

Starting around age three, children become increasingly aware of the environmental and social messages surrounding food. Exposure to the media and to other children adds to this developmental transition. Families report that children suddenly start to request foods by brand name and are increasingly interested in what people around them are eating. For example, young children will request that specific foods be prepared in ever more specific ways. The requested foods may just happen to be identical to the food items regularly packed in a friend's lunch or served at the child's preschool program. For example, three-year-old Alyce sits next to her friend Matthew at lunch. In fact, they have been eating lunch together for the past two years in their child care center. Shortly after her third birthday, Alyce became very observant of the foods Matthew had in his lunchbox. At home, she started to request that the *same items* she admired in Matthew's lunch be included in hers.

At this age, children become very tuned into their food environment and the social settings in which foods are offered. Children observe that special foods—for example, ice cream, cake, cookies, and chips—are served and eaten during celebrations, such as birthdays, other parties, and holidays. The fun and excitement surrounding these events make cake and ice cream taste even more delicious. Buttered popcorn, soda, and hot dogs are frequently consumed at movies and sporting events, two common recreational pastimes in the lives of many American families. These observations and experiences, coupled with children's natural taste preferences for sweet and salty foods, result in these foods becoming favorites. When it comes to vegetables, young children are more likely to hear a parent's complaints about the need to eat "only a salad" or to skip dessert in an effort to manage weight. They observe a family member's regular refusal to eat the broccoli or green beans served at a family meal. The child concludes that these foods are less desirable choices.

Foods that are beneficial to health, such as fruits and vegetables, are frequently offered in a negative, coercive manner. Recognizing the importance of healthy foods, adults sometimes use threats and bribes, such as "When you finish your broccoli, you can have dessert" or "No TV for you tonight unless you clean your plate." Food becomes a reward or a punishment, not a part of healthy living. Sometimes this is what the adult heard growing up; sometimes it results from feelings

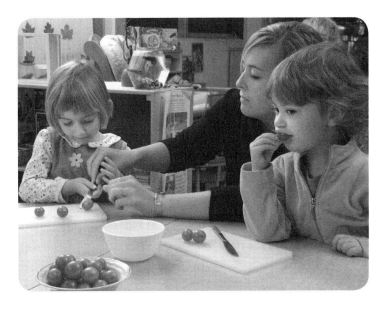

of frustration about the child's food habits. In these scenarios, vegetables become unappealing (Birch and Fisher 1995). The child learns that the adults are in charge of when to eat, what to eat, and how much to eat—and this awareness does not lead to the formation of healthy eating habits. The goal of the Early Sprouts program is for children to choose and enjoy eating healthy foods—even when an adult is not present.

Around age three, children begin to lose their ability to self-regulate the number of calories they consume. As a result, forcing them to eat when they are not hungry diminishes their ability to recognize when they have had enough. Feeling stuffed from eating too much becomes the norm. By late preschool age, children begin to overeat because of environmental and social pressures. For these reasons, it is important to provide young children with age-appropriate food portions and allow them to decide for themselves when they are full. A positive strategy is to invite children to serve themselves small amounts. Assure them that second helpings will be available if they are still hungry after finishing their first portions. When healthy foods are provided, children make healthy choices.

Teachers and family members have the potential to be the most effective role models by offering and enjoying healthy foods in a friendly and supportive environment. To counteract social pressures toward less healthy choices, early childhood educators should provide as many positive social cues as possible about healthy foods. Display your enjoyment of fruits and vegetables. Use healthy foods for celebratory events. Our Early Sprouts classrooms enjoy the program's Carrot Muffins or Butternut Squash Muffins for birthday celebrations. They make vegetable soup or serve veggies with a healthy dip for family events.

It is important to avoid power struggles with young children over food. It is better to focus your efforts on creating positive social environments that support young children in eating the right foods and fostering the development of lifelong healthy eating habits. For example, apple or berry picking with young children can be fun and exciting and provide motivation for children to eat and enjoy the fruits of their labor. Serving raw veggies and low-fat dip as part of a classroom or family picnic can be a successful approach. Planting a vegetable garden can help instill enthusiasm for growing, harvesting, and eating vegetables.

These examples provide suitable ways for offering healthy foods to young children. Here's the bottom line: early childhood educators and families should maintain control over their children's diet, not by engaging in a power struggle but by monitoring the foods that are regularly introduced, available, and served. One of the best ways to do this is to connect children to the sources of food. As you will see, having access to a vegetable garden is a vital part of our approach.

THREE

THE GARDENING APPROACH

CHILDREN CAN BE INVOLVED in growing vegetables in many ways. You can either take advantage of existing resources in your community or plant a garden using whatever space is available. You may want to start small by visiting a local farmers' market or growing a single plant in a clay pot. Or you may want to allocate a portion of your school's play yard for a vegetable garden. Regardless of your budget, you can share the life cycle of plants with your children. Start small, but be adventurous!

Visits to Local Farms, Gardens, and Farmers' Markets

If a school-based garden is not feasible, a visit to a local organic farm or even a neighbor's backyard garden is a rewarding way for children to watch food grow. Children enjoy this experience even more when it is combined with an opportunity to pick and taste the foods they observe growing. You can further reinforce this experience by a visit to a local farmers' market during the harvest season. During this visit, you can help the children recall their farm adventures.

The twenty-four-week Early Sprouts curriculum lasts much longer than the gardening season in many climates (including ours in New Hampshire!). Buying vegetables from alternate sources may become necessary. The Early Sprouts program features vegetables that are readily available year-round. Because the vegetables and the recipes are used as snack or meal items, some of the cost of food supplies will be covered by your food budget. Supermarkets, grocery stores, or natural foods stores may be willing to provide food donations or substantial discounts to school-based nutrition initiatives. Farmers' markets and Community Supported Agriculture (CSA) programs are other great sources of produce. Visit www.localharvest.org to identify local farmers and farmers' markets.

Indoor and Container Gardens

If you are interested in gardening with your preschoolers but lack growing space, you can try indoor growing or container gardening. Both of these options provide children with seed-to-table exposure and an understanding of the origin of their food. Additionally, these methods tap into children's natural sense of curiosity and adventure.

Indoor gardening can extend the growing season for preschool centers located in northern regions. Although indoor gardening has some limits of its own, it can be done, providing a helpful alternative for preschools with limited outdoor space. Careful attention to temperature, pollination, light, and fertilization are required when gardening indoors. For example, leafy crops (including Swiss chard), root crops (including carrots), and tomatoes can all be cultivated indoors. Butternut squash, however, is unlikely to thrive indoors because it needs so much space and has special pollination requirements.

Here are a few tips for successful indoor gardening:

- Purchase vegetable seeds in late spring or early summer: it is often difficult to find seeds in mid to late summer at garden centers. In those months, it is best to order directly from a seed company (see appendix C, Recommended Organic Seed Sources, page 197); select bush beans, small-rooted carrots, Swiss chard, bell peppers, and determinate varieties of cherry tomato seeds or seedlings.

- Place leafy greens and root vegetables in a cool yet bright location (an enclosed sunporch that stays above freezing is an ideal location).

- Locate tomato, green bean, and bell pepper plants in a warmer location with temperatures ranging from 60° F to 70° F; a sunny classroom window may provide a suitable growing environment.

- Build or purchase an indoor growing station; these are an ideal way to start seedlings.

- Lightweight soils are a must for indoor gardening, so do not use outdoor garden soil. Make your own indoor soil mix by combining equal amounts of compost, vermiculite, peat, and perlite.

- Water indoor vegetables daily; small growing containers and dry indoor air cause the soil to dry out quickly.

- Apply a well-diluted liquid fish or seaweed emulsion to indoor plants every other week. (Fish emulsion can create an unpleasant indoor odor.)

- Manually pollinate your flowering plants, such as the tomato, green bean, and bell pepper plants, using a small paintbrush to gently distribute pollen from one flower to the next; this activity provides an ideal opportunity to discuss the important work of bees.

Container gardens enable us to enjoy plants in areas where a traditional garden is not possible. Container gardens require outdoor space with good sunlight but are usually located in small spaces—even a small porch, balcony, doorstep, or windowsill can produce an impressive harvest of vegetables in containers. Large pots, window baskets, hanging baskets, old buckets, wooden barrels, and plant boxes can all be used to grow Early Sprouts vegetables with children. Here are a few tips for successful container gardening:

- Plant your container garden at the same time you would plant a regular garden; after planting, carefully soak the soil with water.

- Water your container garden daily, because small containers dry out quickly; during the hottest weeks of the summer, we suggest watering in both the early morning and evening with a rain wand or a gentle sprayer.

- Select containers that drain readily but retain enough moisture to keep the plants' roots moist.

- Use large containers that hold 20 to 100 quarts to allow for root development and moisture retention.

- Use compost or a high-quality organic potting mix to fill your containers— "soil-less" potting mixes work best. You can also make your own by mixing equal parts of peat moss, sand, and loamy garden soil.

- Place your container garden in a location that provides no fewer than five hours of direct sunlight each day. (Swiss chard can tolerate less sun, carrots will need more sun exposure, and tomatoes, bell peppers, and green beans will need the most. Butternut squash plants can be grown in a large container but will need room outside of the container for the vines to sprawl.)

- Remember that your container garden is mobile. Relocate the containers as the sun changes patterns throughout the growing season; wheels make relocating them easier.

- Fertilizer will be washed away each time you water, so fertilize your container garden frequently. Liquid fish or seaweed emulsions are good basic fertilizers.

Herb Gardens

An herb garden with different textures and smells can interest children. Herbs also add great flavor when you are cooking with your target vegetables. You can plant herbs with your vegetables using a technique known as *companion planting*. Companion planting provides homes for beneficial insects and repels certain pests. Basil and parsley do well with tomatoes, for example. Dill, parsley, and cilantro attract beneficial insects. When a cocoon or chrysalis forms on your herbs, you have a living science lesson in your play yard. Children will watch the transformation from caterpillar into moth or butterfly with wonder.

Play Yard Vegetable Gardens

If space is available, or as your confidence in gardening with children builds, you may want to consider a play yard garden. In this section and in appendix B, Preparing the Garden Site (page 191), you will find lots of information to help you get started on this venture.

GARDEN PLACEMENT

Locating your Early Sprouts garden in the play yard allows you and the children easy and frequent access to the gardens and the vegetables growing there. This proximity makes the garden part of the children's daily lives rather than something exotic and inaccessible. With daily contact, the children will be more actively involved in observing plant growth and in harvesting the vegetables and other plants you grow. The location will depend, of course, on available space, sunlight, access to water, and other property and physical space considerations. Alternate potential locations include lawn or flower beds adjacent to the entrance of your facility, a spot outside the classroom windows for easy viewing during the day, or, for urban dwellers, a rooftop. Designing, constructing, planting, and maintaining your Early Sprouts garden is an exciting process when you embark on the program.

DESIGNING THE GARDEN

Select the best location for your Early Sprouts garden. Start by paying careful attention to which areas of your play yard get the most sun. Most vegetables require a minimum of five to six hours of direct sunlight per day. If you are observing your outdoor space in the winter or early spring, remember to consider the shade that

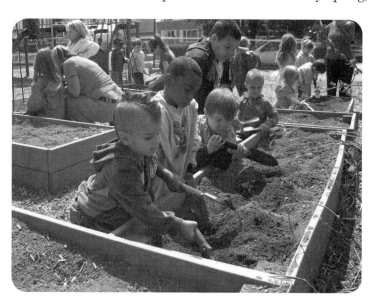

will soon be created by nearby trees. The angle and location of the sun changes with the seasons as well.

An equally important consideration is the location of a water source. This is especially crucial in areas where there is minimal rainfall during the growing season. Be sure all parts of your garden can be watered easily, preferably with a garden hose or sprinkler. Newly planted seeds and young seedlings should be kept moist and require gentle daily watering. Hand watering during the height of summer is very labor intensive. Mulching your garden can help, for you don't want a weekend drought to wither your ripening vegetables!

Also important are accessibility and the positioning of your garden within your play space. The garden should invite children to enter in and explore, yet protect the plants. Other aspects of the play space will need to be considered, such as areas for climbing, digging, running, riding wheeled vehicles, and playing with balls and other outdoor toys. Young children need help remembering when it is acceptable to dig in the garden (while preparing the soil for planting or after harvesting when they pull plants out) and when it is not (while the seeds are sprouting or young plants are growing). Classroom design principles that advise locating active and quiet play spaces in different areas apply here (Curtis and Carter 2003, Isbell and Exelby 2001). For example, you may want to locate one portion of your garden in a high-traffic area of your play yard and another portion of the garden in a more remote location. As you plan the locations, think about how the garden will affect the flow and energy in your play space.

We use raised beds for our Early Sprouts gardens. This allows us to locate the garden beds in the best spots for sunlight, access to water, and play yard design. You may want to use an existing garden area or dig up a portion of your yard to create an open soil bed. This decision requires other considerations. If you plant your seeds directly into an open soil bed instead of into raised beds, pay attention to soil drainage. If you are planting directly in the soil, be sure to have your soil tested for lead and pesticides before you break ground. Take note of what areas of your play yard tend to always be damp and what areas are prone to drying out quickly. Vegetable plants thrive in soil with a balance between draining well and holding some moisture.

Garden soil also needs appropriate nutrients and an appropriate acid-to-base (pH) balance for the plants you select. Soil testing reveals the nature and quality of your garden soil and indicates what you should add to balance your soil ingredients for growing plants (for details, see appendix B, Preparing the Garden Site, page 191).

Although attractive and productive gardens can be created by seeding directly into the soil, we have found several advantages to using raised beds for planting:

- ❦ Drainage: raised beds are designed and built with good drainage in mind
- ❦ Soil temperature: the soil warms faster in the spring and stays warmer into the fall
- ❦ Soil compaction: the soil stays looser because people aren't walking on it
- ❦ Soil composition: raised beds are filled with fertile, weed-free soil
- ❦ Plant spacing: fertile soil allows closer spacing of plants, resulting in higher yield and greater variety per square foot
- ❦ Care and maintenance: the raised height makes it easier to weed the soil and tend the plants

Our Early Sprouts gardens are located in the children's outdoor play spaces. The raised beds, located in boxes built from composite decking, provide excellent protection that minimizes accidental trampling and puts the growing plants close to children's eye level.

The first task in designing your garden is to create a layout that is inviting and welcoming for young children. The configuration should stimulate innovative play. For example, you may choose a layout that resembles a maze. Another option is to take advantage of playhouses located in your play yard and create cottage-style gardens. Cottage gardens are quaint, easily accessible to the playhouse, and take advantage of whatever space is available. Provide a minimum of three feet of space between beds so children can easily run, skip, or bike through them. The garden area can contribute to children's gross-motor development as well as offer them cognitive and creative learning experiences. Raised beds can be used to create an interesting space that will stimulate children's creativity well beyond the growing season.

The total size of your garden will be dictated by the space you have available. Obviously, the larger the garden space, the more plants you can grow. Because Early Sprouts relies on purchasing vegetables through the local grocery store or supermarket during the off-season (for us, the winter months), you don't need to be able to grow everything you will use for the entire program. We believe that having the garden adds to the effectiveness of the program, so do what is reasonable to include some garden space.

Raised beds can be placed on top of surfaces like concrete or wood chips. Each of our current Early Sprouts gardens has its own arrangement, bed sizes, and creative approach to incorporating the garden in the play yard. Here is an example of a layout we have used:

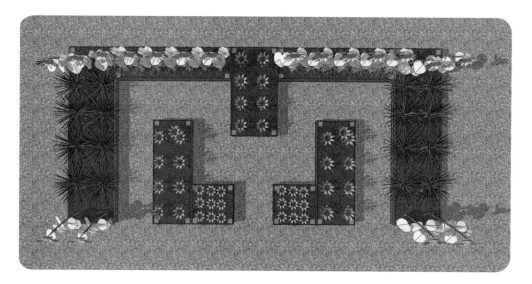

(See appendix B: Preparing the Garden Site, page 191, for detailed information on how to construct garden beds.)

FILLING YOUR RAISED BEDS WITH SOIL

The foundation of organic gardening is well-nourished soil. A fertile soil is a mix of 15 percent compost, 15 percent sand, 70 percent loam, and possibly some lime (depending on the results of a soil sample). You will need enough soil to fill each of the raised beds to within 2 to 4 inches from the top. Organic soil is available through local landscapers and garden supply stores. The ultimate goal is to provide your plants with a nutrient-rich, dark-colored, sweet smelling, crumbly soil full of earthworms. (See appendix B, Preparing the Garden Site, page 191, for more information on soil and soil preparation.)

WHY ORGANIC?

When gardening with young children, you want to make the experience as safe as possible. Conventional gardening frequently relies on harsh synthetic pesticides and fertilizers. Many of these products are toxic. Children can easily get sick when their hands go directly from dirt containing pesticides and fertilizers into their mouths.

Organic gardening does not rely on harsh chemicals and therefore is the preferred way to garden with children. Organic gardening creates a healthy gardening environment by relying on feeding the soil, creating healthy plants that do not need to be fed with chemical fertilizers and pesticides. By choosing to garden organically, you also minimize chemical runoff from fertilizers and pesticides. This runoff often pollutes local drinking water or winds up contaminating lakes, streams, and water treatment plants.

Organic does not always mean nontoxic. Some organic pesticides and fertilizers (derived from plant, animal, or mineral sources) are just as toxic as conventional products. Several organic fertilizers are safe and can be used to supplement the compost and other soil amendments. We recommend liquid fish emulsion and seaweed fertilizers. We suggest avoiding all pesticides when gardening with children and instead (when necessary) hand-picking insect pests from the plants. Marigolds and other companion plants also repel some insects when planted along the garden edge. If you do decide to use an organically approved pesticide, please do so with great care. (Readers can find more information in this chapter's Where to Get Gardening Help section, page 43, and appendix D, Gardening and Vegetable Resources, page 199.)

Growing vegetables organically is a commitment to a sustainable practice in which humans and nature live in harmony. Once you become part of this process, you realize that a few holes or blemishes on your produce or a small reduction in yield are not so bad after all. And the produce harvested from your Early Sprouts garden will be pesticide free and rich in vitamins and minerals.

PLANNING AND PLANTING THE GARDEN

Now that you have prepared your soil, created your garden plan, and purchased your seeds and/or seedlings, you are ready to plant when the weather permits. Just before planting in your already tilled soil, lightly rake your garden beds to create a smooth surface. As you prepare for this step, plan how children and families can assist in planting the garden. Schedule an appropriate date for setting out your garden, depending on your USDA Plant Hardiness Zone.

At this step, the children can become directly involved. They will enjoy digging, sowing seeds, and planting seedlings. They will want to please and will follow clear and careful directions that are developmentally appropriate. Remember that the Early Sprouts garden is primarily a children's garden. Its purpose is for children to learn about vegetable gardening. Some seedlings may accidentally get damaged or seeds may be sown in locations not intended. All of these instances provide opportunities for learning and exploring. (Growing, maintaining, and harvesting each of the Early Sprouts target vegetables are discussed in chapter 6.)

After your seeds and seedlings have been planted, water your garden well. We recommend a rain wand that attaches to your garden hose. The rain wand provides a gentle, yet thorough, watering and allows children and families to successfully assist in caring for the garden.

> **SUGGESTED GARDENING TOOLS (IN CHILD AND ADULT SIZES)**
>
> • Buckets
> • Broad fork to hand-till raised beds
> • Hand trowels and hoes
> • Harvesting baskets
> • Hoes
> • Hoses and sprinklers
> • Measuring sticks and rulers
> • Pruners (kept in a safe location)
> • Rakes
> • Row markers
> • Six-foot bamboo or wooden stakes to stake up tomato and pole bean plants
> • Shovels
> • Thick yarn and scraps from women's hosiery for tying up plants
> • Tiller (hand or electric)
> • Watering cans
> • Wheelbarrow

Maintaining the Garden

Any successful gardener can attest to the importance of garden maintenance. Watering, weeding, thinning, and fertilizing are all critical aspects to caring for your garden to help ensure a fruitful harvest.

WATERING

It is important to water frequently during the early stages of plant growth and while plants are forming and ripening fruits. Plants can become damaged and fruits can be stunted from too little or sporadic watering. At the beginning, the garden should be watered almost daily, unless a substantial late afternoon or evening rain occurs. Children love to help water the garden, although they will need some assistance in reaching all corners of the garden beds. During summer vacations, we recruit families and children to sign up for daily watering shifts.

It is important to provide some basic instructions to help families succeed at this chore. It is considered best for the plants to be watered during the early morning hours or after sunset. If plants are watered with a sprinkler during the heat of the day, their leaves and fruits scorch when watered, and the bulk of the water evaporates rather than seeps into the soil. A drip irrigation system for watering reduces loss through evaporation, but it is costly. To best support the growth of your plants, you want the majority of the water to go into the soil, not directly on the leaves of the plants. Gentle, thorough watering is the best practice here, just as gentle rain supports plant growth without damaging tender sprouts.

WEEDING

As your vegetables grow, so do unwanted garden weeds. Sometimes it appears that weeds grow faster than the desired vegetables! Familiarize yourself with how your vegetable seedlings should look so you do not accidentally pull them during weeding. If the seeds were planted in a row, you can usually recognize that the row plants are not weeds. Try to pull or hoe weeds when they first appear; small weeds are easier to uproot and create less soil disturbance when removed. Placing mulch around your vegetable plants is a great way to control weeds and maintain soil moisture. Organic gardening books provide great advice on selecting specific mulch for various vegetable plants (see appendix D, Gardening and Vegetable Resources, page 199).

THINNING

Typically when planting small seeds, such as those of carrots, young children sow too many. When this occurs, it is important to thin out the sprouts while they are still small. Following the spacing guidelines on the back of the seed packages, remove sprouts until the recommended spacing is achieved. This task requires care so as not to disrupt the roots of the plants you want to remain growing in your garden. (See chapter 6 for tips on growing the Early Sprouts target vegetables.)

FERTILIZING

Mild fertilizers, such as liquid fish or seaweed emulsion, are ideal for organic gardens and are relatively safe for humans. These fertilizers provide nitrogen and other nutrients needed for early vegetable growth. We recommend that you apply liquid fish or seaweed emulsion one week after seeds have sprouted and when the seedlings are transplanted. Follow the directions for dilution and amount on the type of fertilizer you purchase. Here's a rule of thumb: Go light on the application of fertilizer. Too much fertilizer can be more harmful than too little, especially if your soil is well prepared before planting. Be sure to dilute the fertilizer to the appropriate concentration prior to application, because fertilizers are often sold in concentrated form. Heavy-feeding vegetables, such as tomatoes, benefit from regular fertilizer treatments. A monthly dose of a 5-3-3 organic fertilizer can keep them actively growing all season long.

HARVESTING THE BOUNTY

After many weeks of watering, weeding, and watching the garden grow, children will be eager to start picking the fruits—and vegetables—of their labor. Green beans and Swiss chard can be harvested shortly after they first appear. In fact, picking the beans and trimming some of the larger Swiss chard leaves help the plants to produce more. Other Early Sprouts vegetables, such as tomatoes, bell peppers, and butternut squash, require a bit more patience until the fruit is fully ripe. Of course, when gardening with young children, many vegetables will be picked before their peak ripeness, thus providing lots of learning and tasting opportunities.

Using a Cover Crop

At the end of the harvest season, after you have removed all remaining plants, you have a final opportunity to nourish your garden's soil. The warm days of late fall allow you to grow a cover crop. Cover crops replenish soil nutrients diminished during the growing season, minimize erosion (especially important for open-soil gardens), and prevent weed growth. Before planting a cover crop, turn the garden over with a tiller or a spading fork. Level the garden soil with a rake and scatter the cover crop seeds by hand, spreading them as evenly as possible.

Winter rye is an ideal cover crop for cold climates. Be sure to plant the grass at least a few weeks before the ground freezes. In the early spring (three to four weeks before planting your garden), till the cover crop into the soil. Be sure to select a cover crop that is adapted to your region's climate. We suggest consulting with a local organic farmer, a Cooperative Extension gardening expert, or your local nursery staff for specific suggestions.

Rotate the location of your crops annually. Crop rotation is crucial to maintaining healthy soil. For example, alternating the location of your tomatoes and green beans from year to year helps to keep your soil's nitrogen in balance. Each new gardening year brings the joy of planning a new garden layout and experimenting with new varieties of vegetables, flowers, and herbs. Your Early Sprouts garden is a growing opportunity in many, many ways!

Composting

Composting is the microbial decomposition of organic matter under controlled conditions. Put another way, composting turns stinky kitchen food scraps and yard waste into rich, productive soil. Bacteria, fungi, worms, and insects all contribute to creating compost from food scraps, dead plants, and other organic matter into something wonderful. Implementing a play yard composting system helps your garden in several ways:

- Uses food scraps that would normally have been thrown away in the garbage
- Creates nutrient-rich compost that can enrich your garden for the following growing season, contributing to the garden being self-sustaining
- Completes the children's exposure to the cycle of life that your play yard garden embodies so well

(For details about composting, see appendix B, Preparing the Garden Site, page 191.)

Questions of Budget and Funding

The gardening component of your program does not need to be expensive. You can start small with a few bags of seeds, some soil, and a few pots. Or you can spend a few thousand dollars building an elaborate raised-bed garden with a drip irrigation system. The majority of our Early Sprout gardens required an initial investment of $1,000 for materials to build raised beds, acquire soil, and buy garden tools/equipment. Once established, we spend about $75 per year on seeds, seedlings, manure, and other garden enrichments.

GARDEN START-UP BUDGET	
Composite decking	550
Cedar posts	100
Composite decking screws	20
Soil	200
Garden tools	80
Seeds	20
Seedlings	30
Total	**$1,000**

Where to Get Gardening Help

To date, all of our Early Sprouts play yard gardens have experienced great growing success! But occasionally you may need to consult an expert about a particular gardening concern. Most organic farmers are enthusiastic about seeing your garden succeed. They can provide excellent advice on locating and rotating plants, cover cropping, preventing plant disease, and managing pests. We have been fortunate to have an organic grower serve as a gardening consultant from time to time. To get in touch with a local farm, visit www.localharvest.org and enter your zip code to find farmers in your area.

Local Cooperative Extension Service offices employ knowledgeable gardening consultants who can serve as an excellent resource. Be sure to tell the extension consultant that you are growing and managing your garden organically and that children actively participate in gardening activities. This information helps the extension agent assist you in safely involving the children in the garden. The Cooperative Extension Service also trains and coordinates the Master Gardeners program. To achieve and maintain Master Gardener certification, a gardener must complete a designated number of garden-based service hours. You may be able to recruit a Master Gardener to complete his annual service hours in your Early Sprouts garden. Your local garden club is another potential resource for help. Finally, a knowledgeable staff member at a local gardening supply store is another reliable source of gardening advice.

We are not experts at vegetable gardening, but we have found success even with our limited expertise. The good news is that the target vegetables are easy to grow. Good soil, adequate fertilizer, plenty of sun, and sufficient rain augmented by watering in dry climates or months are all you need. The most important things are a positive attitude and a willingness to try. The children will learn about plant care and the cycle of seed to harvest regardless of how many tomatoes or green beans you are able to pick. So relax and give it a try. You can learn new skills through participating in Early Sprouts, as we have. And you will have the wonderful pleasure of fresh-picked vegetables that come from your classroom or play yard garden as a benefit to you and your preschoolers!

^ **FOUR** ^

Preparing Staff
for "Planting" Early Sprouts

THE EARLY SPROUTS APPROACH introduces vegetables through a variety of experiences—gardening, sensory exploring, cooking, and eating. Because one of our major goals is to shift children's taste preferences toward new vegetables, the ways teachers and caring adults introduce the vegetables are vitally important to the success of this curriculum. In this chapter, we share some suggestions to help you prepare for Early Sprouts. Adults are significant and powerful role models for young children. If a teacher doesn't want to try a new food or expresses surprise at a child's interest in eating Butternut Squash Muffins, for example, she is sending a negative message to that child. If the teacher models a willingness to try a new food even when he doesn't like it yet, he is encouraging the child to take a risk and try the food herself.

Chris, a pre-K teacher, shared this anecdote. One of the children in the pre-K class, Rachel, is characterized by her family as being a picky eater. When Chris mentions the Early Sprouts vegetable of the week, the comment is, "Rachel won't like it." Rachel is interested in cooking, however. When the class was preparing an Early Sprouts recipe, Rachel was one of the first children to wash her hands and come to the table. "I could do this every day because I love it," she would say. But she continued to refuse to taste any of the results of the cooking activities. One day, Chris sat down next to Rachel at the snack table. Rachel repeated that she didn't like Butternut Squash Muffins. Chris reminded her that they had prepared them together and asked Rachel if she had tasted one. Rachel glowered and said nothing. Chris then took a bite of a muffin and said "Mmmm, this is yummy." Rachel was hungry. She lifted the muffin to her nose and sniffed it, stuck out her tongue and licked it, broke off a tiny crumb and slipped it into her mouth. Chris just kept eating, quietly observing to see would happen next. Eyes opening wide, Rachel took another bite, and then another. "Wow, I really like these!" She consumed four mini muffins before snacktime was over. While Rachel is still hesitant to try new foods, Chris's gentle modeling and encouragement were effective in getting this child to take a risk and try a new food.

The language we use is very important in influencing children's thought processes and shaping their responses to new experiences. If we describe a food as "bad tasting," "strong flavored," or "yucky," we are inviting children to reject that food. If, however, we use words that describe the process of learning to like a food, acknowledging that everyone does not like the same foods, we support them in learning to like foods that aren't familiar. In the Early Sprouts program, we have adopted the following phrases to describe our responses to a new food:

- "I like it a lot!" We use this to describe a strong positive preference for the food.

- "I like it a little bit." We use this phrase to describe a neutral response to the food.

- "I don't like it yet." We use this to describe a negative or unfamiliar reaction to the food.

We find that children readily adopt this language. Three-year-old Jayne's teacher reported that she had not tried the Veggie Burger recipe during the classroom cooking experience. At home, when she and her mom were preparing this same recipe as part of the Family Recipe Kit, Jayne stated that she didn't like veggie burgers at school, but now she liked them a little bit. When we use these phrases to describe our reactions to foods, we teach children that taste preferences can change. Children understand that with repeated opportunities, they can learn to like new foods.

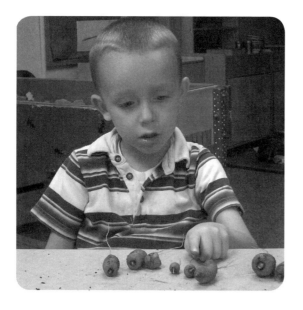

Because some adults are unfamiliar with gardening and/or cooking, support and training for staff are important to the success of Early Sprouts. If the teachers haven't learned to like vegetables yet, eating the recipes can be intimidating. We have developed some suggestions to help teachers, assistants, and other adults involved with preschool children become positive role models. (See Early Sprouts Tasting Suggestions for Teachers, page 51.) Positive adult role models influence children's health and nutrition in beneficial ways. By offering children multiple opportunities to participate but not requiring or pressuring them to taste or eat the vegetables, we provide the ideal conditions for behavior change.

Preparing to Garden

Gardening provides the opportunity to care for plants and learn more about the life cycle of the natural world. Many urban and suburban dwellers do not observe vegetable gardening in their communities, although rooftop, backyard, and community gardens exist in these environments. Fortunately, many experienced people across the country and in your community can assist with this aspect of the Early Sprouts program. Bookstores and garden shops sell books that offer tips and techniques for a range of gardeners. (See chapter 3, Where to Get Gardening Help, page 43, and appendix D, Gardening and Vegetable Resources, page 199, for more information on gardening.)

> In his book *Seedfolks* (2004), Paul Fleischman describes the joy that a community garden can bring to isolated and lonely city dwellers. Preschool children would enjoy this book as a read-aloud.

The most important attributes that a gardener needs are an open mind and a willingness to get dirty. (Even then, gardening gloves can help with dirty hands!) Plants teach us about the cycle of nature—when things thrive and when they wither and die. You learn firsthand what ingredients plants need to survive, such as soil, water, light, and temperature appropriate to each plant. Select plants that are easy to grow for your area, and give gardening a try. If you are unable to plant a garden, visit a local farmers' market to purchase seasonal produce. Who knows? You may find someone there who would be willing to grow some vegetables for your classroom!

Preparing to Explore

The Early Sprouts curriculum includes exploring, cooking, and eating selected vegetables. Each component of the program is purposeful and has clear learning objectives. When children explore a vegetable, they learn about it through their senses and engage in discovering the vegetable's properties. They describe its characteristics, observe, and document their responses. They follow directions and work with others to create a recipe. They ask questions and experiment to find answers. Each week of the curriculum includes a sensory exploration.

These qualities—learning through their senses, discovering properties and characteristics, observing and documenting, following directions, asking questions, and experimenting to find answers—are also used to describe the importance of play as a tool for young children's learning. We advocate a play-based curriculum and believe that children learn many things most effectively through play, as opposed to teacher-directed instruction (Bredekamp and Copple 1997). Despite these similarities, in the Early Sprouts curriculum we do not say we are playing with food. We don't want to confuse children, who are often told not to play with their food at mealtimes. We describe the open-ended experiential learning as "exploration" and invite children to explore and taste the vegetables.

Preparing to Cook

Cooking with preschool children can be one of the most rewarding aspects of the classroom curriculum. Young children are naturally curious about the world around them. Cooking activities provide the opportunity for them to engage directly in the real work of preparing food. The Early Sprouts recipes will add to your repertoire of classroom cooking activities.

Many cookbooks provide ideas for cooking with children. What makes Early Sprouts unique is its focus on cooking healthy recipes that feature vegetables as main ingredients. While carrot cake and zucchini bread recipes do include vegetables, their main flavors come from other ingredients. We do not try to hide the vegetables or disguise them. Instead we highlight them in the preparations and often in the name of the recipes to foster positive recognition of vegetables as important foods in healthy diets. This approach is effective, as seen in the following example. Four-year-old Ethan commented, "I like honey, and I know I'll like Honey Glazed Carrots." Now that he has eaten them, he knows that he likes carrots too.

All our recipes have been field-tested in numerous classrooms by teachers who love to cook "from scratch" and by others whose main cooking experience is to warm food in a microwave oven. The recipes were developed with the developmental levels of preschool children in mind. Their directions include strategies to involve the children in the cooking process. We have compiled some general cooking principles here that will assist you when cooking with a group of children. (You will find all of the recipes in chapters 8 through 11.)

PLAN AHEAD

First, always review the recipe, gather the ingredients and tools, and mentally prepare yourself before cooking. A cooking experience can be messy and challenging, so knowing and planning the steps in advance are important to the project's success. It is best if you try the recipe ahead of time so you feel more confident in how to proceed, just as it's a good idea to read a story to yourself before you read it aloud to a group of children. Determine the desired group size for the particular recipe as part of your preparation. Children may or may not stay for the entire process, so think about how to involve newcomers along the way. It is best if children feel able to choose to participate, observe, or leave the cooking activity. Self-determination is important in all educational programs, because we want to nurture independent children who can make choices and decisions.

Teachers must model careful hand washing and hygiene when cooking. Children and adults should wash their hands thoroughly before handling any ingredients, after licking or touching other items, and again when they leave the activity. Children are encouraged to taste the vegetables; however, they may need adult guidance to put an ingredient that has been handled or licked into the compost container, not back into the mixture. Remember to sanitize work surfaces and equipment regularly. Simple common sense, clear observation, and gentle reminders on the part of teachers go a long way. Soon the children will help each other be careful with their shared food.

USE OF TOOLS

When you provide developmentally appropriate cooking tools, preschoolers can shred or chop ingredients. Serrated plastic knives are useful for chopping, and plastic graters promote ease in grating softer ingredients, such as cheese, while preventing children from damaging their skin. Provide each child with an appropriate tool, a container for collecting the chopped or shredded items, and a clean working surface, such as a plastic or paper plate or a cutting board. Precutting the vegetable or other ingredient into smaller amounts will allow many children to participate and give each of them a manageable portion for the task. The goal is to foster involvement and a feeling of success. Because the recipes are designed for use with young children, precise chopping isn't required.

Some of the recipes call for a small electrical appliance, such as a blender or food processor. With such tools and appliances, safety is paramount. Children can fill the container while the appliance remains unplugged and then operate the power switch with adult supervision. Place your appliance on a counter so that the cord does not present a hazard in the classroom's walkways. Children can stand on stools or platforms to reach the controls. Likewise, with careful setup and supervision, preschool children can assist with cooking that requires a heat source, such as a hot plate, microwave, convection or conventional oven, or electric skillet. If these appliances are not available in the classroom, you can arrange for the children to visit the kitchen facility to observe this part of the cooking procedure.

Sounds and sights of the ingredients being chopped or whirled together are very exciting for young children. The smells that come from baking inspire everyone to want a taste. As young scientists, children are interested in observing the changes that occur. Carrots are transformed to small shreds for use in Carrot Oatmeal Cookies. Chunks of butternut squash combine with milk, banana, and yogurt to become Banana Squash Smoothies. Wet and dry ingredients combine and fill muffin cups, then bake and turn golden brown as they change from batter to Confetti Corn Muffins.

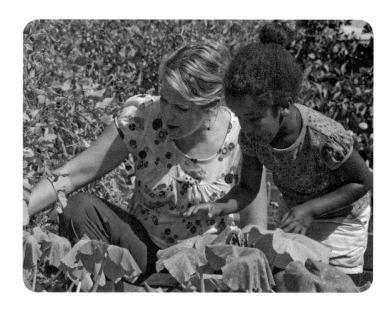

INVOLVING CHILDREN

One of the goals of the cooking component of the program is to involve children in the real work of preparing and cooking food. Plan specific ways that children can actively participate. Preschool children can't wait for a long time, and just watching does not sufficiently engage most of them. Plan how you will manage turn taking so that many children have an opportunity to participate. Rotate the turns quickly and provide a clear description of what each child should do. An explanation, such as "First Jonas will stir while we count to five, then Truc will go next, and then it will be Ingrid's turn," provides clarity for the children. Such instruction contributes developmentally appropriate structure and guidance for preschoolers.

Young children are very capable of filling containers and dumping them out. You can harness this ability by providing a container of the appropriate size (that is, a measuring cup or spoon) and having the child fill it with the ingredient. Two cups of cornmeal can be divided into four half cups, allowing four children to be involved in the measuring. When the exact amount of a specific ingredient is important, you can have children measure the amount into a separate container. Doing so prevents too much of a minor ingredient, such as salt or baking powder, from accidentally being dumped into the mixture. Children can be taught to crack eggs and dump them into a small bowl for hand beating prior to adding them to a batter. Liquids, such as canola oil, can be poured into the measuring spoon by an adult, while the child carefully holds it over the bowl.

Many of the Early Sprouts recipes, such as English Muffin Pizzas with Homemade Tomato Sauce, Cheddar and Chard Quesadillas, and Green Bean Wontons, have children assemble individual portions. Children prepare the ingredients and make the snack or lunch by following the directions you provide. A picture chart provides a model for them to follow while making individual portions of pizza or wontons, which then are shared with their friends at mealtime. Other recipes, such as Bell Pepper Fried Rice or Chinese-Style Green Beans, are made in a large quantity and then divided into portions at serving time. Children can help prepare ingredients by measuring or chopping, adding them to the mixture, and stirring to combine all the ingredients.

Some children eagerly participate in all cooking activities. They want to make several of an individual item or contribute to preparing the entire recipe. Other children come for a few minutes and help, but then move on to another part of the classroom. Still others merely observe the process and procedure. These variations may reveal a child's temperament, learning style, or developmental readiness to join a group. However, each child is also being exposed to the vegetable because it is part of the classroom curriculum. All should be invited to taste the finished product when the food is served.

Preparing to Taste at Snack or Meals

One challenge we faced at the outset of Early Sprouts was motivating teachers and families who might not enjoy vegetables, who "don't like them yet." Early childhood professional guidelines recommend that adults sit with children during meals and snacks (Harms, Clifford, and Cryer 2005). Early Sprouts adds to this expectation by describing how to model willingness to try new foods. Because adults are such powerful role models for young children, and children's food choices are influenced by the social and emotional aspects of the environment (Birch, Zimmerman, and Hind 1980), teachers and parents or guardians should be willing to try a portion of the Early Sprouts food when it is served. If you don't like the food, be discreet about your response and allow yourself the opportunity to "learn to like it" too.

The Early Sprouts recipes can be used as snacks or as part of a meal, depending on the needs and focus of your program. Some of our Early Sprouts programs prepare lunch for the children. These programs have their cook prepare an additional portion of the featured recipe, in addition to the amount the children prepare, so everyone can eat it at lunch. (We include portion information in the recipe section to guide your planning in this regard.) Allow children to serve themselves an amount they think they can eat or are willing to try. This provides them with a sense of control over their food choices. Children can be responsible for how much food they want to eat and whether or not they eat at a given time. Adults take responsibility for the quality of food, its nutritional value, and for making it available at appropriate times (Satter 2000).

It is important that you do not offer an alternate food when serving one of the Early Sprouts recipes. The presence of an alternate food implies to the child that she probably won't like it and that you expect her to eat something else instead. (The exception, of course, is when a child is allergic to one of the ingredients in a particular recipe.) Because preschool children are often naturally picky eaters, this guideline is critically important. Young children eat when they are hungry, and they aren't always hungry on a program's or group's schedule for meals and snacks. During the meal or snack, encourage children to take a tiny

EARLY SPROUTS TASTING SUGGESTIONS FOR TEACHERS

- Always eat a portion of the Early Sprouts recipe; children will be more willing to try the recipe if you are eating with them.

- Invite children to serve themselves from a common bowl by taking one scoop from it; when a child has finished eating the first scoop, offer her a second helping.

- Be a positive role model; be adventurous about trying new things and encourage the children to do the same. Try to encourage all children to try at least one bite of the recipe.

- If you like the recipe, share your enthusiasm and positive comments; if you do not like the recipe, please be discreet (do not openly criticize the food).

- Compliment the children on the recipe—many of them participated in making the snack! Thank them for their hard work making delicious food.

- Ask the children to explain how they made the food (for example, ingredients, stirring, measuring); they will be proud of their hard work and the recipe.

- Talk about pleasant things and discourage the children from talking about unpleasant topics or openly criticizing the food offerings.

taste, and explain that they need to find out whether they have grown to like the food. Remember that by using this vocabulary—"You don't like it yet" or "I like it a little"—to describe their response to the recipe, you are teaching children that it is normal for food preferences to change and that they can learn to like new foods.

Keep the table conversation pleasant, and praise the effort and involvement of the children who helped prepare the recipe. Use descriptive phrases, and ask questions about the process—for example, "You chopped a lot of bell peppers for this recipe!" or "How did you make this delicious tomato sauce?" This approach offers children the opportunity to explain what they did, which reinforces their experience and demonstrates what they remember about it. As Aristotle said, "Teaching is the highest form of understanding." When children can teach us what they have learned, they truly understand it.

(For more ideas and information, see appendix E, Books about Cooking with and for Children, page 201.)

The Early Sprouts curriculum helps teachers learn more about nutrition and gain skill in cooking as a component of the curriculum. The benefits for children are significant, and teachers and families can potentially improve their own nutrition and health. As preschool teacher Karen said, "Participating in the Early Sprouts curriculum has been a most rewarding teaching experience. I have always had an interest in gardening with young children, but the Early Sprouts curriculum took my interest and commitment to a new level." The Early Sprouts program defines how to make gardening and nutrition part of the curriculum all year round. We are pleased to share our actual curriculum—the sensory explorations, recipes, Family Recipe Kits, and strategies—for adapting and adopting to your location.

Bon appétit! ¡Buen provecho! Enjoy your meal!

FIVE

INVOLVING FAMILIES

A S EARLY CHILDHOOD EDUCATORS, we believe families are the primary teachers in their children's lives. Families have a significant impact on children's development in all areas—physical, cognitive, social, and emotional. They are even more vital when it comes to young children's dietary preferences and habits (Birch and Fisher 1996). The nutrition and food environment in children's homes substantially affects children's health and the formation of their eating habits. The home can serve as another place for positive exposure to vegetables and healthy eating, so we have developed effective strategies for involving families.

Through participation in the Early Sprouts program, families learn ways to involve their children in food preparation at home. The Early Sprouts curriculum becomes more effective with family involvement through communication, participation, events, and feedback.

An Accepting Approach

When families purchase the food, prepare the meals for children, and convey messages about health and nutrition, what they say and do affects their children significantly. Perhaps for this very reason, discussing food and nutrition with families of young children can be very challenging.

Many families with young children have limited time to prepare balanced meals. They may not have extensive knowledge about healthy food choices, and they are confronted with a lot of contradictory information about children's food. Fast-food restaurants provide toys as rewards for purchasing meals. Food products are marketed specifically to children, regardless of their nutritional profiles. Some home recipes recommend hiding healthy foods in baked goods. Many families may not understand that children can be taught to eat a range of foods through calm, repeated opportunities to try them. When new foods are not presented that way, children resist trying any new foods.

Family members, especially adults, also often feel vulnerable to comments about what their children eat or what they feed their children. They worry about being judged for their children's behavior, food preferences, or family values around food. Working families sometimes find that feeding their children is one area of family life where they feel some control, especially when children are spending a large portion of their waking hours in early childhood education settings. Although these reactions are typical (Galinsky 1987, Rudney 2005), each family experiences them differently, making a "one size fits all" response impossible.

Information about servings and portion sizes that are recommended for preschool children will help families relax about how much food their children consume. The rate of physical growth as seen in height and weight gain slows down during the preschool years, as compared to infancy and toddlerhood. Therefore, the amount of food eaten will often plateau and sometimes decrease during this period. We want to support families so they don't persuade their children to eat more than is needed. It is also important to encourage children to eat foods that provide nutritional balance and establish healthy eating habits for life. Families need to be reminded that offering children healthful foods is the goal.

We recognize that food is a sensitive issue for many adults, personally and as parents or guardians, and that their own responses to eating behaviors will shape the children's future eating habits. Picky eaters can be a challenge, and family members may worry that their children won't get enough to eat if they don't have their favorite foods on a daily basis. Sometimes adults haven't developed a preference for healthy foods themselves and are vocal about their dislike for certain foods. Children naturally absorb these attitudes and decide they don't like the foods either. Sometimes family members who are dieting inadvertently influence their children

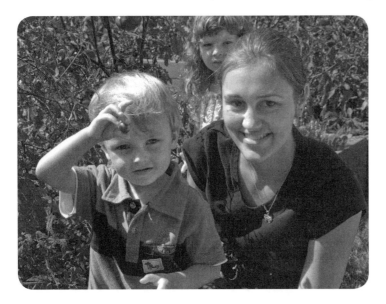

by saying "I can only eat salad" in a disparaging tone of voice, reinforcing the concept that eating salad is a punishment or a sacrifice. Most of us have used candy or ice cream to praise accomplishments or soothe hurt feelings and disappointments. This can result in a child associating comfort or celebrating exclusively with sweets. Because we understand these challenges, we don't want to add stress around food. Rather, we want to support families to make healthy choices that are simple and don't take a lot of time. The Early Sprouts program provides alternatives by encouraging families to foster healthier eating habits and increase vegetable consumption.

Focusing on the positive and encouraging small steps to improve children's food intake is relatively easy. Suggest foods to add to their diet, mentioning the corresponding health benefits. Recommend lunch and snack foods that are easy to prepare but don't necessarily come in elaborate packaging. For example, children enthusiastically eat baby carrots or fresh fruit slices with yogurt dip. These snacks provide families with choices and help them avoid the snack aisle in the grocery store. The Early Sprouts Family Recipe Kits provide families with recipe ideas to prepare and eat at home with their children. State and national standards emphasize healthy nutrition (NAEYC 2007) and can provide support to teachers who are providing families with guidelines for their child's food intake. Sharing this knowledge with families in the form of newsletter articles is another strategy teachers can use to support families who are working on their children's eating habits. We find that positive suggestions result in better changes than a list of prohibited foods.

Our accepting approach with families takes into account the fact that behavioral change takes time. We use encouraging and positive language in all of our written materials as well as when we meet with families. We try to focus on what they might *do* to increase the nutritional value of a meal or snack. We don't want families to feel criticized, so we do not focus on what they might *not* be doing for their children. We recognize that taking baby steps toward a healthier lifestyle produces more realistic and achievable results. We want families to be partners in teaching and learning about foods and nutrition through the Early Sprouts curriculum.

Family Communication

The families of the children participating in the Early Sprouts curriculum are kept well informed throughout the entire program. At the outset, families receive information that describes the Early Sprouts program in detail (see sample letter, page 56). We include permission forms for their children to participate in the food tasting and for us to photograph children involved in the program (see sample permission form, page 57). Additionally, each newsletter we send to families has a column describing the Early Sprouts activities. These brief articles describe classroom vignettes, provide photos, and share teachers' comments about children's responses to the curriculum (see sample newsletter article, page 58). A family bulletin board with photos and narrative describing children's involvement keeps families aware when on-site (see suggestions for bulletin board narratives, page 59). Communication boards located in classrooms announce the vegetable, sensory exploration, and recipe planned for each week. Families receive helpful tips for positively engaging their children while preparing food and trying new recipes together. (Recipe tips for cooking with children are included in the Family Recipe Kits in chapter 12.)

Sample Letter to Families

Dear Families,

Our Preschool Center is implementing an exciting nutrition and garden-based program, *Early Sprouts: Cultivating Healthy Food Choices in Young Children*. A vegetable garden is now located in the play yard. All children enrolled in the preschool classrooms and their families are invited to participate.

It isn't always easy to get children to eat the right foods. Let's face it: you can serve your children all the vegetables in the world, but if they don't like them, they aren't going to eat them. The intent of the Early Sprouts program is to increase children's preference for vegetables through the experience of helping to grow, prepare, and taste featured vegetables.

Starting in fall and continuing through spring, children will be invited to participate in weekly in-class, food-based activities that feature vegetables and stress their importance in maintaining health. Children will explore vegetables using all of their senses and assist in the preparation of healthy snacks using produce gathered from the garden (when in season).

Each week, children will also be invited to help prepare and take home a weekly Family Recipe Kit containing all necessary ingredients to prepare the week's featured vegetable at home. We ask your help in assisting your child to prepare the featured food item. This way you, too, can participate in this exciting project with your child.

Finally, you will be invited to participate in food-based activities throughout the year. This will allow you to experience the Early Sprouts program firsthand. Please let us know if you have any questions or comments as we learn together.

Sincerely,

Early Sprouts: Cultivating Healthy Food Choices in Young Children

PERMISSION TO USE PHOTOGRAPHS

Early Sprouts photos are frequently needed—they're used primarily for grant requests, public relations materials, and publicity purposes. We are requesting permission to use photographs of your child for the purposes listed below. All photographs will be approved by the center's director prior to use and children's names will not be included in the use of the photographs.

I give permission for photographs of my child, _____,
to be used in the following ways as <u>initialed</u> by me below:

_____Center public relations materials

_____Local, regional, and national newspapers/publications/other
media

_____Early Sprouts Web site

_____Photo displays for professional presentations and grant
proposals

_____Photo displays for community presentations

Signature of Parent/Guardian: _____

Date: _____

Classroom: _____

This form is valid for the duration of your child's Early Sprouts experience unless a new form is completed.

Family Participation

FAMILIES IN THE GARDEN

Families are invited to participate in garden planting and care. Weekend seed or seedling planting parties can provide a way for all to see the garden cycle begin. Families can help water and weed the garden during times when the program may be closed or the weather is particularly hot or dry. This activity keeps them involved with Early Sprouts throughout the growing cycle and provides an additional investment in the curriculum. When this work is shared with other families, participants also gain the benefit of social time with children and family members.

EARLY SPROUTS THEMES FOR FAMILY EVENTS

Family events enrich the life of the classroom and build a bridge between home and center life that supports children's learning experiences. Using the vegetables and recipes as a curricular theme, the Early Sprouts program can offer opportunities for families to participate in centerwide events during the year.

To celebrate the beginning of the year, try hosting a pancake breakfast using the Early Sprouts recipe for Butternut Squash Pancakes. Breakfast at the center provides a convenient way for families to come early and learn about the classroom because they don't have to eat breakfast at home first. Children make the batter and families take a few extra minutes to eat with their child at the morning arrival time. Children really enjoy showing their families the parts of the classroom that are special. Teachers have the opportunity to meet families and become more acquainted. What a fun and nutritious way to start the day!

A popular children's story based on an old folk tale provides inspiration for one special family event. Our preschool classrooms host a Stone Soup luncheon for families during the harvest season. Integrating the Early Sprouts program, the children prepare recipes, such as Confetti Corn Muffins with bell peppers and Pita Pocket Pizzas with Swiss chard. They make the Stone Soup using the six target vegetables. In addition to the food preparation, children send home invitations, make place mats and other classroom decorations, set the table, and host their families for the harvest celebration. Rhonda, a teacher who has prepared a Stone Soup luncheon for years, reports, "Children actually eat the soup now. We talk about the vegetables and they connect them to our garden and to Early Sprouts. There is more discussion at home about what vegetable to bring

---

(SAMPLE NEWSLETTER ARTICLE)
SEPTEMBER EARLY SPROUTS NEWS

The children in the preschool classroom have been busy harvesting vegetables from the play yard garden over the last two weeks. On Tuesday, several groups of children went to the garden to pick green beans and brought them back to the classroom to wash and explore. The children discovered the seeds within the seedpod when they dissected the vegetable. On Thursday, the children cooked delicious Chinese-style green beans using tamari, which is a wheat-free soy sauce. Many children hadn't eaten tamari before and discovered they enjoyed it! We hope you enjoy making this green bean dish with your child at home this week.

in. The kids really feel ownership of the soup and want to eat it all." Families join their children at the lunch hour to share a nutritious meal prepared by the children. Both families and children are very proud of this accomplishment.

The Early Sprouts program can also be extended to the community through field trips. Three- to five-year-olds are becoming aware of the world around them. They are curious and want to participate and understand their community environment. In our area, field trips to an orchard to pick apples provide a connection to the natural world, fun for families and children, and a harvest of healthy food for all. Participating in a local community garden or shopping at the farmers' market increases families' ability to build community relationships. Each of these field trips reinforces the foundational principles of the seed-to-table experience for the children. We try to encourage families to provide children with experiences in the community by organizing family field trips to a local farm in the summer and an orchard in the fall.

There are many ways to include the Early Sprouts program in event planning. For example, include family potlucks and family cooking nights that feature Early Sprouts target vegetables and recipes; parent/guardian-teacher evenings can be focused on the Early Sprouts nutrition approach. These events provide further opportunities for families to learn about the program and nutrition in a relaxed, meaningful way.

GATHERING FEEDBACK FROM FAMILIES

The Early Sprouts program aims to increase nutritional experiences and ideas for families. For that reason, linking back to families and asking for feedback is very important. Gaining honest feedback helps us to improve. Through a series of family surveys, focus groups, and questionnaires, we learn a great deal about what is or is not working from families' perspectives. We ask families to describe their experiences, share changes that occur at home, and make suggestions. Then we use this information to make changes and respond to specific issues. Each year we make an improvement plan based on family feedback because we want the Early Sprouts program to remain vital and personally engaging to families. Attending to family concerns helps us increase family involvement and meet the needs of families.

For example, families suggested changes to recipes that were too complicated or did not offer sufficient child participation. We also adapted the frequency and timing of the Family Recipe Kits in response to family feedback. (You'll find a sample feedback form to include with the Family Recipe Kits in chapter 12 and focus group and survey information in chapter 13.)

BULLETIN BOARD SUGGESTIONS

At the start of the school year, the Early Sprouts bulletin board was used to describe the program by its major themes:

• Gardening

• Sensory Exploration

• In-class Cooking

• Packing Family Recipe Kits

The teachers collected photos from the previous year to depict each of these themes. A narrative describing each component was included.

When family members have time to reflect and share their insights, they are more interested in the program. They become more fully aware of what foods their child eats on a regular basis. They can think about the small additions they might make to their child's diet. They start to reflect on what foods are available in the refrigerator and cupboards at home. They can plan the next steps to extend Early Sprouts into the life of their entire family. Families have been overwhelmingly positive in their response to the program. This is because we are providing suggestions for foods to add to their family meals, not criticizing their current dietary choices.

Family involvement in the Early Sprouts program is one of our goals. When families are involved, we know the potential for healthy eating in the home increases. We believe that positive change in our nation's health will occur when change occurs in each family. We have learned that when we provide a variety of experiences with vegetables, children become interested in exploring vegetables. By communicating carefully and respectfully with families, we support children's interest being incorporated in their home. When we convey knowledge about nutrition, healthy foods, and behavior change, families respond. Our care and attention to this connection between the curriculum and the family helps us know Early Sprouts will have a lasting impact.

SIX

THE EARLY SPROUTS
TARGET VEGETABLES

ALTHOUGH EARLY SPROUTS IS PRIMARILY FOCUSED on nutrition education, the program also contributes to the development of knowledge and vocabulary related to plants, vegetables, and nutrition for both adults and children. Four-year-old Thomas announces to the group at lunch, "I'm eating a nice nutritious banana." While most children won't remember the nutrients gained from eating green beans or cherry tomatoes, they do absorb the terminology about plants and nutrition when the adults around them use correct terms. Five-year-old Nina is drawing a picture of the squash plant. She says "I used a lot of light green. There's lots of buds on this plant. That's what they're called—buds." We don't expect you to memorize the nutrients in each vegetable, but we hope you will use your newfound knowledge and become more curious about the foods you eat.

At the outset of the Early Sprouts project, we chose six vegetables as our target vegetables. We focused the garden, sensory explorations, recipes, and family involvement around these six vegetables. Our research shows that children's willingness to taste these six vegetables increased and that it also increased for other "novel" vegetables not targeted by the actual curriculum. Of course, not every child or family grows to like each of these vegetables, but the original six are a good place to begin your adventure into Early Sprouts.

Here is some basic information about each vegetable: how it grows, its nutritional contribution to healthy eating, and fun facts about it. The vegetables are listed in the order in which you will see them presented in the curriculum. We begin with tomatoes because they are familiar and have a "sweet" taste, making them a good place to start the program.

Tomatoes

BACKGROUND INFORMATION

Tomatoes are one of the most popular garden vegetables. There are hundreds of varieties of tomatoes, ranging from very small, pea-sized ones to fruits as large as two pounds each! Their shapes vary from round like a globe to those of plums, pears, or grapes. Tomatoes also come in a variety of colors, including red, purple, orange, pink, green, and yellow. Tomato plants are typically categorized as indeterminate or determinate. Indeterminate varieties produce more fruit than determinate varieties. Because indeterminate varieties grow taller and taller throughout the summer, they require trellising or other support. Determinate varieties do not grow as tall as indeterminate varieties and need less support. They also tend to produce the majority of their fruit over a short period of time. Determinate varieties are good choices for container gardening. If you have limited garden space, we definitely recommend you try to make room for cherry tomatoes, one of the smaller varieties of tomato. They are easy to grow, very prolific, and often sweeter than standard slicing tomatoes. In our Early Sprouts gardens, cherry tomatoes are a very popular play yard snack. The Sun Gold cherry tomato is an orange variety and the sweetest tomato we have found!

PLANTING AND CARE

Tomatoes like the heat and grow best when seedlings are transplanted into warm soil. Be sure to add lots of compost prior to planting because tomatoes require nutrient-rich soil. After the risk of frost has passed, plant your tomato plants 2 to 3 feet apart in the garden. Bury the seedlings as deeply as you can, leaving at least 2 inches of the top of the plant out of the ground. This creates a thicker stalk and a hardier plant. At the time of planting, place a large stake next to each tomato plant to provide support once the plant grows taller. Staking tomato plants decreases the risk of disease and increases productivity. As the tomato plants grow, tie them to the stakes or trellis. Use thick yarn or scraps from women's hosiery to attach the plant to the support system. Water your tomato plants regularly. As they grow, remove any side shoots or suckers to keep the plants from becoming too full and tall. Pruning the top leaves during the late season helps redirect the plants' energy from growing leaves to producing fruit. Until the plants stop flowering, apply a monthly dose of liquid fish or seaweed emulsion.

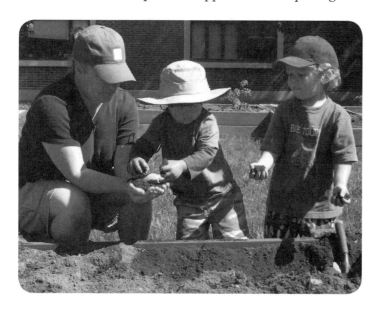

HARVESTING

Tomatoes have the best flavor when they are allowed to fully ripen on the vine. That's why garden-fresh tomatoes are so special. Tomatoes will continue to ripen off the vine, but they will not have the rich, summery tomato flavor of fresh-picked fruit, so try to pick tomatoes only when fully ripe. If there is a threat of frost, you may want to cover your plants or harvest your tomatoes before they are fully ripened. Fruits off the vine will ripen best in a shady, warm location.

HOW ARE THEY COOKED?

Most people are familiar with cherry tomatoes as a garnish in a green salad. Cherry tomatoes can be eaten right off the vine or with a savory dip as a snack. Fresh tomatoes also make great salsas that can be spicy or mild, depending on the additional ingredients you select. Ketchup has a tomato base, and sun-dried tomatoes start as fresh tomatoes too. Tomatoes are featured in many cuisines—for example, in gazpacho, marinara sauce, pizza, tomato juice, soups, stews, sauces, and stir-fries.

FUN FACTS

- Tomatoes are a good source of vitamin C and potassium.

- Tomatoes are believed to have originated in South America and were first cultivated in Central America and Mexico.

- When tomatoes were introduced to Europe, in some northern regions they were confused with a poisonous plant known as deadly nightshade, and assumed to be poisonous; they were grown only for decoration until the nineteenth century.

- The tomato is scientifically considered a fruit, but in 1893, the U.S. Supreme Court ruled that the tomato was a vegetable so it could be taxed.

- A tomato is more flavorful when stored at room temperature, so please don't refrigerate your tomatoes.

- China is the country that grows the most tomatoes, while the states of California and Florida grow the most tomatoes in the United States.

- Relatives of the tomato include potatoes, bell peppers, and eggplants.

For more information, visit www.growtomatoes.com.

Green Beans

BACKGROUND INFORMATION

Green beans are part of the legume family. The green in green beans does not refer to their color, but to the fact that they are harvested and eaten before being totally ripe. Different varieties of green bean seeds include bush beans and pole beans, as well as different colors of beans. Bush bean plants are short and compact, making them an ideal harvest height for young gardeners. Bush beans are ready to harvest in fewer than 60 days and can usually be harvested only twice. Pole bean plants can grow to be more than 10 feet tall, but they take up less space because they twist and turn around their support. A pole bean play yard teepee is popular with young children. Pole beans continue to produce over a much longer period and have a higher yield than bush beans. Young gardeners enjoy planting the large bean seeds, which sprout quickly. It is almost guaranteed that you will end up with an abundant harvest. Green bean seeds are also ideal for indoor growing and can assist with cycle-of-life discussions.

PLANTING AND CARE

Beans are an easy plant to grow and are not particular about their soil conditions. They grow on vines in warm and sunny environments. The seeds should be planted directly in the garden. Plant your seeds after the risk of frost has passed and the soil has started to warm. Plant seeds 1 to 1½ inches deep. For bush beans, sow the seeds every 2 to 3 inches in rows that are 18 to 24 inches apart. Sow pole beans 4 inches apart next to a trellis or around teepees. You can plant as many as 6 seeds around each pole. Thin pole bean plants to 6 inches apart in trellised rows or to a total of four plants around each pole. When pole bean plants are 6 to 8 inches high, you may need to guide them to the trellis or nearest pole.

HARVESTING

Green beans take about 60 to 75 days to mature. Pick the beans when their firm pods contain fully formed (but not dried-out) seeds. You can also do a taste test to discover the size when your variety of beans has reached its peak flavor. Beans need to be picked frequently for the plants to continue producing additional fruits.

HOW ARE THEY COOKED?

Green beans may be roasted, steamed, sautéed, or eaten raw. Wash fresh beans thoroughly and then snip the stem end with kitchen scissors. Green beans can be cut into 1- to 2-inch lengths, sliced lengthwise (French style), or left whole for cooking, dipping, and eating. The color of purple-podded green beans changes to dark green when cooked, but yellow beans remain yellow. Green beans are featured in many cuisines, especially in stir-fries, soups, and salads, and as side dishes. They can be garnished with sauces or lightly steamed. They are easy to freeze.

FUN FACTS

- Green beans are a good source of vitamin A, vitamin C, and folic acid.
- Beans are believed to have originated in South and Central America; different varieties have been cultivated around the world since ancient times.
- In the folktale Jack and the Beanstalk, a magical beanstalk grows tall enough to take the boy, Jack, into the clouds, where he finds a giant.

- Beans are one of the "three sisters" of companionate planting developed by the native peoples of North America using maize, beans, and squash. The maize or corn plants formed the pole for the bean vines to climb and provided shade for the squash. The beans added nitrogen to the soil, which nourished all of the plants. The squash grew around the base of the corn plants and served as mulch, protecting the beans and corn from weeds and preserving moisture in the soil. Because squash vines can be prickly, they also discouraged animals from coming close and eating the plants.

- Green beans are also called *string beans* or *snap beans*. In early varieties, the green bean had a "string" down the length of the bean that was tough and had to be removed, hence the name *string bean*. Modern varieties have been bred to grow without the heavy, fibrous string.

- Yellow beans are sometimes called *wax beans*.

- Dried beans provide protein and can be eaten instead of meat.

- China, India, and Brazil grow a lot of beans, including green beans, lentils, and dry beans.

- A recipe called Fifteen Bean Soup has (you guessed it) fifteen different kinds of beans in it!

- Relatives of the green bean include pinto beans, black beans, and kidney beans.

For more information, visit www.greenbeansnmore.com/index.htm.

Bell Peppers

BACKGROUND INFORMATION

The name *bell pepper* refers to the shape of the fruit of the capsicum plant, which comes in both sweet and hot varieties. Bell peppers, also called *sweet peppers*, contain

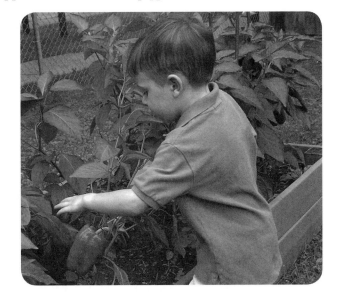

a recessive gene that eliminates the spicy capsaicin found in other hot or spicy pepper varieties, such as cayenne, jalapeño, and tabasco. Bell peppers are available in a wide variety of colors, shapes, and flavors. The edible part is the mature fruit of the plant, which usually features either three or four lobes. If your location has a long growing season, bell peppers will continue to ripen and change color to yellow, orange, or red, depending on the variety. Be sure to check the length of time needed to grow each variety of pepper, and select one that will do well in your area.

PLANTING AND CARE

Bell peppers flourish with fertile soil, plenty of water, and warm weather. Peppers grow best when transplanted into the garden as seedlings. Plant and space them 18 inches apart once evening temperatures are consistently above 50° F, usually one week after the last expected frost date in your area. Fertilize with a dose of liquid fish or seaweed emulsion at time of transplanting, and continue to fertilize monthly. Be careful not to overfertilize, or you will end up with lots of leaves and very few peppers. Most pepper plants eventually need to be supported by a sturdy stake. Be sure to provide plenty of water while the peppers are growing to ensure a sweet, moist, and thick-fleshed fruit. Peppers plants are ideal for container gardening.

HARVESTING

You can begin to harvest peppers during their green phase after they reach a usable size. If peppers are left on the plant to ripen, they not only become sweeter but also change color. The fully ripened yellow, orange, and red bell peppers are sweeter in taste and higher in vitamin content. Picking peppers regularly stimulates the plant to produce more peppers.

HOW ARE THEY COOKED?

Bell peppers can be served raw or cooked. Cut around the top of the pepper to remove the stem and seeds. Slice it in half, remove the remaining seeds and white membranes, and then slice, dice, or cut pieces in any size to suit your recipe. Bell peppers are typically roasted, sautéed, or baked (for example, as stuffed bell peppers). Bell peppers can be used in stir-fries, soups, and muffins.

Note: Hot peppers require special handling to avoid skin burns from prolonged exposure to capsaicin. We use only sweet peppers with young children.

FUN FACTS

- Bell peppers are a good source of vitamin A, vitamin C, vitamin B$_6$, and potassium.

- Peppers were first domesticated in Central and South America; archaeologists have found evidence of cultivated chili peppers in Ecuador from more than 6,000 years ago. Bell peppers are now important to cuisines in Asia, Africa, Europe, and the Americas.

- Bell peppers are directly related to all types of hot peppers.

- The spice we call *black pepper* or *peppercorn* comes from a different plant species and is not related to the sweet or hot pepper.

- Many types of hot peppers are grown, dried, and used to season foods all over the world.

- Paprika is made from grinding dried sweet red bell peppers.

- Chilies (hot peppers) can be dried easily and hung on strings. These strings of peppers are called *ristras* in Spanish.

- Other relatives of the bell pepper include potatoes, tomatoes, and eggplant.

For more information, visit www.urbanext.uiuc.edu/veggies/peppers1.html.

Swiss Chard

BACKGROUND INFORMATION

Swiss chard is fun and easy to grow. It grows quickly and can be harvested earlier than some of the other Early Sprouts vegetables because we eat the leaf and the stalk, as opposed to the fruit of the plant. Chard is a member of the beet family and is grown for its succulent, mildly flavored leaves. It is similar to spinach in taste, though some consider it to be slightly more bitter. It comes in several varieties, including Ruby, which features bright red stems, and Bright Lights, which has a rainbow array of stalk colors. We suggest growing several different varieties because the range of colors is very appealing to children. Bright Lights chard is known as *rainbow chard* in our play yard gardens.

PLANTING AND CARE

Leafy greens, such as chard, need nitrogen-rich soil to grow. Add compost prior to planting and apply fish or seaweed emulsion every few weeks throughout the growing season. Swiss chard seeds can be directly sown into the soil two to three weeks before the last expected frost. Sow the seeds ½ inch deep every 1 to 3 inches in rows 12 inches apart. Chard seeds take 5 to 10 days to germinate. Thin plants to 6 inches apart once their leaves are 4 to 6 inches long. These early shoots are a tender and delicious addition to an early season salad. Be sure to water your chard plants frequently to ensure optimal growth and to prevent bolting. (*Bolting* is a gardening term used to describe a plant that prematurely produces flowers and seeds before its edible parts can be harvested.) Chard is a hardy plant and can tolerate mild frosts.

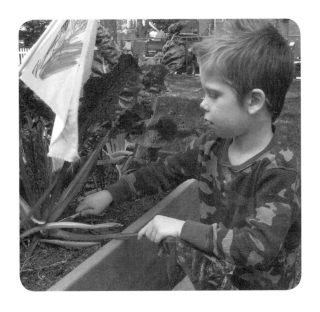

HARVESTING

Harvest chard leaves whenever you are ready to use them after they are large enough to eat. Pick off the larger outer leaves first so the new, centrally located smaller leaves will continue to grow. Chard is a prolific plant and provides lots of edible leaves. For the freshest leaves, harvest the chard just prior to eating or cooking, because it does not refrigerate well. Remember to wash your chard well to remove any sand or soil from its crevices.

HOW IS IT COOKED?

The washed leaves of chard can be eaten cooked or raw. Chard can be used in place of spinach and sautéed in a small amount of oil or steamed until just tender. When added to soups, pizza, rice, or pasta, chard adds color, flavor, and nutrients. Although the leaves are the usual ingredient in recipes, you can also slice the stalks into small pieces, sauté them as you would celery, and add them to stir-fries, soups, or sauces.

FUN FACTS

- Chard is a good source of vitamin A, vitamin C, vitamin E, vitamin K, folic acid, zinc, calcium, iron, magnesium, and potassium.

- Chard was valued as a medicine in ancient times in the Mediterranean region and can be allegedly traced to the Babylonian hanging gardens. Aristotle wrote about red chard in the fourth century BCE, so we know it has been grown and harvested for a very long time!

- Chard got its common name from the *cardoon*, a Mediterranean vegetable related to the artichoke. Its thick stalks look like those of chard.

- Swiss chard is grown in Switzerland but did not originate in this part of Europe, where people call it *Mangold* if they speak German or *blette* if they speak French.

- Cooks in Europe usually prefer to cook the stalk of the chard and not the leaves; in the United States, we usually cook the leaves and not the stalk.

- Relatives of Swiss chard include beets, mustard greens, kale, and spinach.

For more information, visit www.whfoods.com/foodstoc.php, www.cliffordawright.com, and www.justhungry.com.

Carrots

BACKGROUND INFORMATION

Carrots are relatively easy to grow and come in a variety of shapes, colors, and sizes. They are root vegetables and grow underground. Although carrot seeds take a long time to germinate and can be challenging to impatient young gardeners, the joy that comes with harvesting the season's first carrots makes them a rewarding garden treasure. Carrots can easily last into the late fall and even early winter. In warm climates, carrots can be stored right in the ground without added protection. In cooler climates, carrots can be stored in the garden under a thick layer of mulch (for example, 7 to 8 inches of straw). Families will be amazed when their young children report harvesting carrots from the play yard garden following the winter's first snowfall.

PLANTING AND CARE

Carrots thrive in raised-bed gardens. They grow best in cool, loose, weed-free, regularly watered soil. You can plant carrot seeds one to two weeks before your last expected frost. If your soil is dense, select a short, robust variety of carrot. While these may not resemble the grocery store carrot in length, they more than make up for it in sweetness. Rocks, sticks, and other obstacles interfere with the carrots' growth, so remove them. Plant the seeds every ½ inch in rows that are 6 inches apart. After the seeds have been spread, cover them with ¼ inch of soil. Carrot seeds can take up to three weeks to germinate and sprout. Because carrot seeds are so tiny, exact spacing is difficult, so you will need to thin carrot sprouts when they are about 2 inches tall. Initially thin the plants so they are 2 inches apart. About two or three weeks later, thin the carrot plants again to approximately 4 inches apart. When the tops are 5 to 7 inches tall, apply a dose of liquid seaweed or fish emulsion. Sometimes the roots of the carrots begin to expose themselves above the soil line. Covering the root tops with soil prevents them from turning green and tasting bitter.

HARVESTING

Harvest timing depends on the variety of carrot. Be sure to check your seed package for an estimate of maturity time. For sweet-tasting carrots, harvest the carrots after the soil is cool. Their light green, feathery stems and leaves help indicate when the carrot roots are mature and ready for harvesting. Carrots easily survive a few light frosts. Harvest the largest carrot plants first so smaller plants can further develop. The best way to harvest carrots is to rock them back and forth, pulling up on the stems' base near the top of the root. Carrots store well in a root cellar or other cool location.

HOW ARE THEY COOKED?

Carrots can be enjoyed raw or cooked. They get their orange color from beta-carotene and have more beta-carotene than any other vegetable. Steaming, baking, and roasting are great ways to cook carrots. Carrots can be sliced crosswise as coins for stews or puréed for soups. Grated raw carrots are delicious in salads, on sandwiches, and baked in muffins. Carrot juice is another popular way to serve carrots.

FUN FACTS

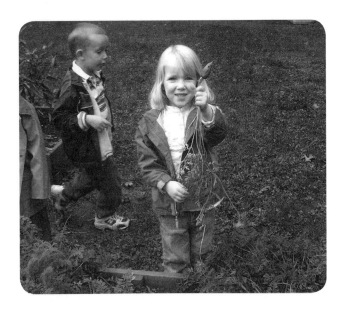

- ❦ Carrots are a good source of beta-carotene and vitamin C.

- ❦ Carrots were first cultivated about 5,000 years ago in Central Asia and Middle Eastern countries, such as Afghanistan; in ancient times, they were recognized more for medicinal uses than for their culinary benefit.

- ❧ Queen Anne's lace is the flower of the wild carrot. Carrots are part of the *Umbelliferae* family, named for their umbrellalike flower clusters.

- ❧ In England in the seventeenth century, women used carrot leaves as decorations for their hats.

- ❧ Carrots were grown by the early colonists in Massachusetts and Virginia in the 1620s.

- ❧ The baby carrots found in supermarkets are actually longer carrots that have been peeled, trimmed, and packaged. True baby carrots are harvested early and look like miniature mature carrots.

- ❧ In Portugal, carrot jam is a delicacy; British cooks like to use carrots in puddings.

- ❧ Relatives of the carrot include dill, fennel, and parsnips.

For more information, visit www.carrotmuseum.co.uk and www.farmdirectcoop.org.

Butternut Squash

BACKGROUND INFORMATION

Squash belongs to the same plant family as gourds and consists of two varieties: summer squash and winter squash. A form of winter squash, the butternut squash has a vaselike shape and a sweet, nutty taste similar to that of the sweet potato. Squash plants grow their fruit on vines with large trailing leaves, stems, and flowers. The fruit of the butternut squash has yellowish-tan skin and edible orange flesh. When ripe, the flesh turns an increasingly deeper orange and becomes sweeter and richer. The tough skin and dense flesh of the butternut squash fruit make it ideal for storing in a cool, dry area.

PLANTING AND CARE

Be sure to plant squash in a location that has space for long creeping vines. Similar to tomatoes and peppers, squash plants flourish in heat. Plant squash seeds after the danger of frost has passed. Add compost to the soil before planting the seeds because squash are heavy feeders. Sow four seeds per foot in rows that are 3 feet apart. Cover seeds with 1½ inches of soil. After they have sprouted, thin plants to 18 inches apart. Fertilize monthly with liquid fish or seaweed emulsion. Pinch off the fuzzy ends of winter squash once the fruits have formed to help them grow larger and ripen.

HARVESTING

Just prior to the first winter frost, harvest your butternut squash. Squash are ripe within 70 to 120 days of planting. You should be unable to pierce the rind with your fingernail. The fruit should be its expected deep color. Leave a 2-inch stem on each fruit. Eat squash with any blemishes first because they will be more prone to rot while in storage. Properly stored squash can last for several months.

HOW IS IT COOKED?

Raw butternut squash has a hard thin skin that is difficult to peel. It is much easier to peel a cooked squash. First, slice the squash horizontally across the very top and bottom so the vegetable has a flat surface. Then cut it in half lengthwise. Remove the seeds, place the flesh facedown in a shallow dish of water, and bake at 350° F until the flesh is tender. Alternatively, cut the squash into smaller pieces, remove the skin and seeds, and then steam or boil the pieces on the stovetop. Use little water to avoid losing flavor and nutritional value. The cooked squash flesh can be added to soups, muffins, and sauces, or puréed and eaten as a side dish. Squash flesh can also be eaten raw. Peeled and grated, uncooked squash is delicious in salads and as a substitute for grated, uncooked carrots. Cooked and puréed squash freezes well.

FUN FACTS

- Butternut squash is a good source of vitamin A, vitamin C, potassium, folic acid, calcium, and magnesium.

- Indigenous populations in South America cultivated different varieties of squash between 8,000 and 10,000 years ago.

- Squash was one of the three sisters, along with corn and beans, used by native people in North America (see Green Beans section for more about this companion-planting technique).

- Squash blossoms are edible; try them in salads or nibble them from the plant.

- Other types of winter squash include Hubbard, buttercup, acorn, and spaghetti squash.

- When you cook spaghetti squash, the flesh separates into ribbons or strands that look like spaghetti!

- In Australia, butternut squash are called *butternut pumpkins*.

- Decorative gourds, the inedible cousins of squash, are used as musical instruments in Africa, Asia, and South America.

- Relatives of the butternut squash include cucumber, delicata, zucchini, and pumpkin.

For more information, visit www.extension.iastate.edu.

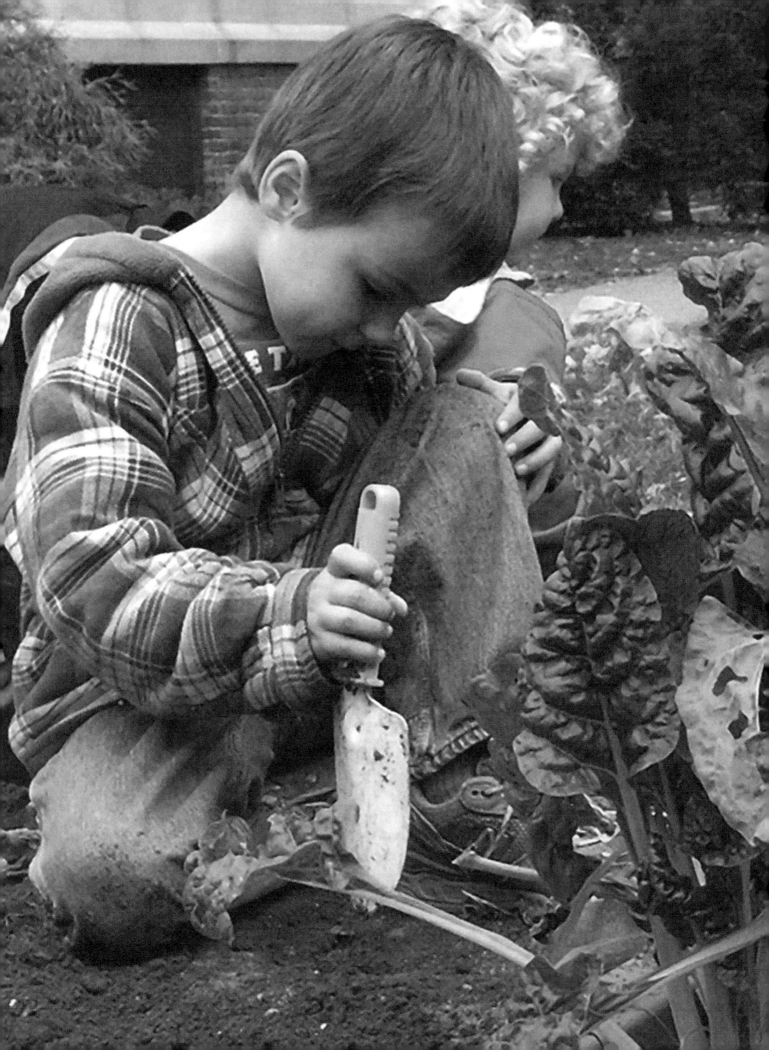

Part 2

TENDING EARLY SPROUTS
Week *by* Week

⌒ SEVEN ⌒

INTRODUCTION TO THE CURRICULUM

THE TWENTY-FOUR-WEEK EARLY SPROUTS curriculum provides simple experiences based on children's innate abilities to be curious, to observe, to wonder, and to explore. The sensory exploration activities and cooking activities are meant to last about 30 minutes to 1 hour on two days of the week. Programs that offer varied enrollment slots often repeat the sensory exploration and cooking activities two times a week so all children have a chance to participate. For instance, on Tuesday and Wednesday children explore the vegetable, and on Thursday and Friday they cook the recipe. While this structure offers more exposure to the vegetable and varied participation from children, it is not required.

We designed the activities for five or six children at a time with children moving through the activities as they desire during choice time. By exploring through the senses, preschoolers are able to smell, touch, see, hear, and taste the vegetables several times over many weeks. Children are guided through the Early Sprouts sensory experiences best when teachers are engaged and excited by the program and value open-ended activities, ask pertinent questions, and build on each child's prior experiences.

We intentionally repeat the structure of the activities over the twenty-four weeks throughout the curriculum:

- First, children are invited to participate in a sensory exploration activity supported by guiding questions by the teacher.
- Next, children cook a healthy recipe featuring the week's vegetable and then eat the prepared recipe.
- Finally, children assist in packing a Family Recipe Kit to extend the experience into their homes.

This structure expands children's observation skills over time and deepens their understanding of the vegetables. The activities are designed to guide children through exploration of each vegetable in a consistent manner so they begin to rely on a predictable progression of experiences. The series of questions teachers ask, the methods of exploring each vegetable, and the possible outcomes for each activity are planned to help children anticipate what might come next. We find this teaching approach is never boring for the children but instead inspires them to expand on their learning in more creative ways because they are comfortable with the process. It also gives teachers familiarity with the content and allows them to be more spontaneous rather than to teach to the book.

A learning environment rich with developmentally appropriate content and appealing materials promotes experiences that are meaningful and purposeful to young children. Literacy, science, mathematics, social studies, and the arts form the content of the classroom and when presented appropriately can instill lifelong interests and successful school experiences. For young children to understand concepts and make connections, they must engage in learning processes that promote investigation, application, communication, and representation (Copley 2000) and handle actual materials to make sense of their ideas. They also need to join with their peers and problem solve together.

Real-life experiences, such as using kitchen tools and preparing food, offer children opportunities to delve into the history of food and the use of simple machines instead of electric appliances. Most children enjoy doing the work of the adults around them, such as using knives, peelers, and graters. They make sense of their world while they engage in the world of adults. Today many of us don't hand-grate carrots, dehydrate tomatoes, or slowly slice open a bell pepper and investigate the insides. Early Sprouts provides the opportunity to slow down and actively engage children in exploring and experiencing selected vegetables.

The Curriculum's Sequence

The curriculum sequence is designed to help teachers move through the twenty-four weeks with ease. We have developed four themes based on the garden cycle:

1. Bringing in the Harvest: The Garden Activities (chapter 8)

2. Harvest Time Is Coming to an End: Bringing the Garden Indoors (chapter 9)

3. Putting the Garden to Sleep: Indoor Winter Activities (chapter 10)

4. Spring Is Coming: Seeds and Planting Activities (chapter 11)

Within the four themes, we include these elements:

- Purpose and objectives
- Six sensory exploration activities with accompanying cooking activity
- List of supplemental activities to enhance the Early Sprouts' integrated approach

You can easily integrate this curriculum into the preschool classroom. Through-out the year, you can incorporate activities in literacy, mathematics, science, and the arts into your curriculum. We have made a few suggestions for additional activities in each of the four themes of the program. Because the curriculum is defined as two 30-minute to one-hour time blocks per week, we do not assume that all your curriculum development will revolve around Early Sprouts. We offer several thematic ideas as starting points for an integrated curriculum. Note as you work with these activities over time the children begin to incorporate what they are learning to other areas of their play.

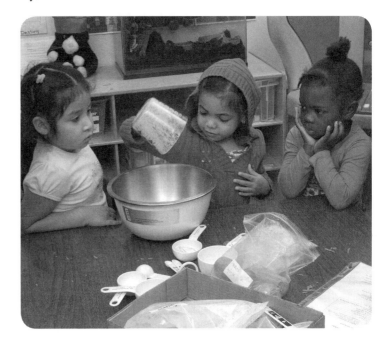

Our Early Sprouts themes begin with the harvest season, typically the time of the year considered the end of the gardening cycle. To bring the vegetables to children in a tangible form at the beginning of the program makes the most sense. While children are involved with garden preparation and planting, the Early Sprouts curriculum focuses on children eating the six target vegetables. The curriculum, therefore, reflects our mission of offering ample opportunities with the actual vegetables.

Call to Action

At the end of each week's cooking activity, you have a perfect opportunity to reinforce the learning by giving a "call to action." The call to action can vary some-what week to week, but always follows the same four steps.

1. Congratulate the children for their excellent work preparing the recipe.
2. Discuss the target vegetable and its characteristics and attributes. This might include such things as color, shape, texture, taste, and smell. It could also involve comparing the vegetable in different states—raw,

dried, and cooked. You might also ask the children about what they learned about in the sensory exploration activity.

3. Encourage the children to eat the target vegetable (or a similar vegetable) at home this week.

4. Remind the children that this week's Family Recipe Kit will include all of the ingredients to make the recipe at home. Finally, encourage the children to help their family prepare the recipe and enjoy it.

The call to action gives you and your students an opportunity to reflect on the week's activities and to carry that learning home.

Materials Needed

Having the right materials easily accessible is one of the critical components of creating an effective classroom environment to support young children's learning. When the classroom is organized and the materials are well prepared, children typically move through the flow of classroom activities easily. Each time the materials are organized ahead of time, the teacher is better positioned to focus on the important task of engaging with children. The materials listed in this section are those Early Sprouts teachers have found most useful.

MATERIALS NEEDED FOR THE SENSORY EXPLORATION ACTIVITIES

- ❦ Blender
- ❦ Bowls in small and large sizes for food collection
- ❦ Child-sized knives, such as flatware or plastic knives
- ❦ Child-sized kitchen scissors to be used only for cooking projects (that is, separate from art use)
- ❦ Colander for washing vegetables
- ❦ Cutting boards in small and large sizes
- ❦ Dehydrator, if available
- ❦ Food processor
- ❦ Grater
- ❦ Plastic gallon-sized bags
- ❦ Plastic airtight containers
- ❦ Trays and aluminum pie tins
- ❦ Vegetable brush for washing vegetables
- ❦ Vegetable masher
- ❦ Vegetable peeler
- ❦ Waxed paper or parchment paper

ADDITIONAL ITEMS NEEDED FOR THE COOKING ACTIVITIES

- Baking sheets
- Ladle
- Large mixing spoons
- Measuring cups and spoons
- Mixing bowls
- Muffin tins
- Oven mitts
- Portable skillet
- Serving cups and plates
- Spatulas
- Whisk

Many of the items listed are nonessential but help make work easier. The dehydrator, for example, is not essential because an oven can be used, but the dehydrator uses less energy, is smaller, and doesn't interfere with using the oven for other purposes. Families or local merchants might be willing to donate some equipment for this program. Other items might be substituted, such as a masher for butternut squash instead of a food processor. Hands, rather than child-sized kitchen scissors, can be used for tearing chard.

You will find the Early Sprouts program is easy to move through sequentially, though it takes time to learn all of its components. Teachers tell us repeatedly what a pleasure it is to observe the children progress from knowing to understanding the vegetables and cooking techniques and, most important, from refusing to taste anything to tasting all the vegetables. When you embark on this journey, you fully embrace the role you play in the lives of children! Taking these small and simple steps toward healthy eating habits will serve you and the children for a lifetime.

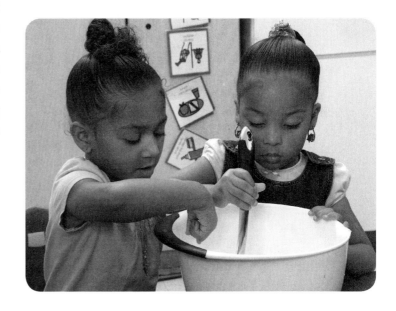

~ **EIGHT** ~

Bringing in the Harvest
The Garden Activities

WEEKS 1–6

GOING TO THE GARDEN each time a vegetable is introduced truly brings an experience of wonder to the children. Imagine a child discovering a full-grown squash on the ground, pulling a carrot from the soil, or happily running toward the many colors of the rainbow as she notices for the first time all of the grown chard. The children often meet these discoveries with awe. They discover how their care and tending of the plants has created the food that they are about to eat. Through handling and exploring, they learn about the different parts of the plants that are edible. They begin to gain an understanding of the seed-to-table concept that the activities promote:

- Identification of the vegetable and its parts
- Recognition of the edible and inedible parts of the plant
- Investigation and examination of the vegetable
- Introduction to descriptive vocabulary
- Taste of the vegetable

Tomatoes

ESTIMATED TIME: 30 MINUTES TO 1 HOUR

PURPOSE

**To provide children with a beginning harvest experience
as a culmination of the growing season,**

❧ Go to the garden with a group of children and locate the tomato plants. Discuss the planting, caring, and growing cycle as a reminder to the children.

❧ Demonstrate how to pick a tomato and give children an opportunity to harvest the tomatoes.

> ❧ What does *harvest* mean? What part of the plant are we picking? What did we do to help this tomato plant grow?

To investigate tomatoes using kitchen tools,

❧ Gather children around a table and provide them with cutting boards and child-sized knives. Remind children that the tomatoes have been washed. Give children opportunities to cut and scrape the tomatoes.

❧ What do you notice about the skin of the tomato?

❧ What do you notice about the inside of the tomato? How do the different parts of the tomato smell, taste, and feel?

For this activity, you will need these items:

❧ 5 or 6 child-sized knives

❧ 1 bowl of cherry tomatoes, enough for 2 or 3 tomatoes for each child

❧ 5 or 6 small cutting boards

❧ Large bowl to collect the tomato pieces

PROCEDURE

1. Children wash their hands and sit at the table. When all children are sitting, teacher hands out the knives. Children use the knives safely to cut tomato pieces.

2. Teacher(s) assists children, as needed.

3. Teacher(s) asks children to place the tomato pieces in the large bowl.

4. If children are interested, let them taste the tomatoes and discuss their texture and taste.

Remind children to wash their hands again if they want to resume cutting tomatoes.

5. Clean up.

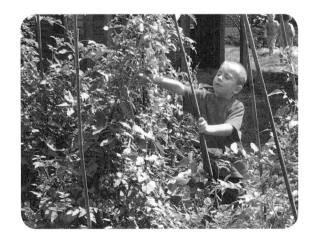

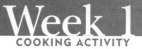

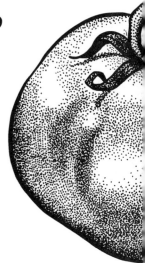

Cherry Tomatoes with Honey Mustard Dip

ESTIMATED TIME: 20 MINUTES

RECIPE
Yields 18 servings
For this recipe, you will need these items:

FOOD INGREDIENTS
2 pints of cherry tomatoes
½ cup low-fat nonfat plain yogurt
2 teaspoons spicy brown mustard
2 teaspoons honey

SUPPLIES AND EQUIPMENT
Measuring spoons
Medium mixing bowl
Spatula
Cutting boards
Plastic or flatware child-sized knives
Mixing spoon
Small dipping cups or bowls,
    one per child

PROCEDURE

1. Wash the cherry tomatoes, slice them in half, and set them aside.

2. Measure and place the yogurt, mustard, and honey in the medium bowl.

3. Stir the honey mustard dip ingredients until they are well mixed and smooth.

4. Using the spatula, pour the dip into small dipping cups or bowls.

5. Enjoy the cherry tomatoes dipped in the honey mustard dressing.

Suggested Ways to Involve Preschool Children in Cooking Activity:

🌶 Have children wash their hands and sit or stand around the activity table.

🌶 Announce, "Today we will use cherry tomatoes from the garden to make Cherry Tomatoes with Honey Mustard Dip." Have children help you rinse the tomatoes in the sink.

🌶 To prepare the tomatoes, children can practice cutting cherry tomatoes using child-sized knives. Finish any incomplete cutting yourself.

🌶 To combine the ingredients, older children (four- to five-year-olds) can measure the ingredients and younger children (two- to three-year-olds) can pour them into the bowl.

🌶 Children can take turns stirring the dip until it is mixed well.

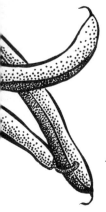

Green Beans

ESTIMATED TIME: 30 MINUTES TO 1 HOUR

PURPOSE

**To provide children with a beginning harvest experience
as a culmination of the growing season,**

- Go to the garden with a group of children and locate the bean plants. Discuss the planting, caring, and growing cycle as a reminder to the children.

- Demonstrate how to pick the green beans and give children an opportunity to harvest the beans. Show the children how to snap the stem off. Explain that the stem connects the green bean to the vine. The stem transports minerals and vitamins from the plant to the bean.

- Encourage the children to feel the outside of the pod. Explain that this is a container that holds the bean seeds inside.

- Ask the children what else could fit inside such a small pod. Snap the beans in half and invite the children to remove a few seeds. Explain that inside the beans are seeds. Ask the children what else can grow from a seed.

- What part of the plant are we picking? What did we do to help these bean plants grow?

To investigate green beans using kitchen tools,

- Gather children inside and provide them with cutting boards and child-sized knives. Remind children that the green beans have been washed. Provide children the opportunity to cut and dissect the green beans.

- What do you notice about the parts of the green bean? What do you notice about the inside of the green bean? Can you eat all the parts? How do the different parts of the green bean smell, taste, and feel?

For this activity, you will need these items:

- 5 or 6 child-sized knives
- 1 bowl of green beans, enough for 2 or 3 beans for each child
- 5 or 6 cutting boards
- Large bowl to collect the cut green beans

PROCEDURE

1. Children should wash their hands and sit at the table. When all children are sitting, the teacher hands out the knives. Children use the knives safely to cut bean pieces.

2. Teacher(s) assists children as needed.

3. Teacher(s) asks children to place bean pieces in the large bowl.

4. If children are interested, have them taste the green beans and discuss their texture and taste. Remember to have children wash their hands again if they want to resume cutting green beans.

5. Clean up.

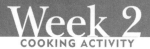

Chinese-Style Green Beans

ESTIMATED TIME: 35 MINUTES

RECIPE

Yields 18 servings

For this recipe, you will need these items:

FOOD INGREDIENTS

1½ pounds green beans

2 tablespoons unsalted butter

2 tablespoons low-sodium tamari
   (wheat-free soy sauce)

2 teaspoons lemon juice (½ squeezed lemon)

8 cups water

SUPPLIES AND EQUIPMENT

Nonstick skillet

Measuring spoons and cups

Long wooden spoon

Serving bowl

Colander

Large pot

PROCEDURE

1. In a nonstick skillet, melt the butter over low heat on the stovetop. Place a large pot of water on another burner and bring it to a boil.

2. Clean the green beans and remove their stems. Snap the beans in half.

3. When the butter has melted, remove it from the heat. Using a wooden spoon, stir in the tamari and lemon juice. Set aside.

4. Add the green beans to the boiling water and boil for 5 minutes or until tender.

5. Turn off the heat and drain the green beans in a colander.

6. Add the green beans to the butter/tamari mixture and gently toss the beans to combine them with the sauce.

7. Serve family style and enjoy!

Suggested Ways to Involve Preschool Children in Cooking Activity:

🌱 Have children wash their hands and sit or stand around the activity table. Announce, "Today we are going to make a recipe called Chinese-Style Green Beans."

🌱 Introduce and briefly describe the origin of each ingredient for the recipe as you place it on the activity table.

🌱 To prepare the green beans, children can wash them, snap off their stems, and snap the beans in half.

🌱 To combine ingredients, older children (four- to five-year-olds) can measure and younger children (two- to three-year-olds) can pour ingredients.

🌱 As always, remember to keep children away from all sharp cutting utensils, electrical devices, and hot food and surfaces at all times!

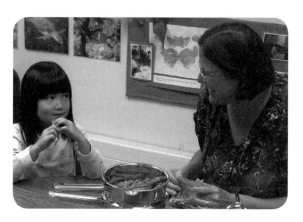

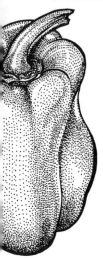

Bell Peppers

ESTIMATED TIME: 30 MINUTES TO 1 HOUR

PURPOSE

To provide children with a beginning harvest experience as a culmination of the growing season,

🌶 Go to the garden with a group of children and locate the bell pepper plants. Discuss the planting, caring, and growing cycle as a reminder to the children.

🌶 Demonstrate how to pick the bell peppers

and give children an opportunity to harvest the peppers.

🌶 What part of the plant are we picking? What did we do to help these pepper plants grow?

To investigate bell peppers using kitchen tools,

🌶 Gather children inside and provide them with cutting boards and child-sized knives. Remind children that the peppers have been washed. Give children opportunities to cut and dissect the peppers.

🌶 What do you notice about the parts of the pepper? What do you notice about the

inside of the pepper? Can you eat all the parts? How do the different parts of the bell pepper smell, taste, and feel? List some words to describe the inside of the pepper.

🌶 Introduce how to dice a bell pepper in preparation for this week's cooking activity.

For this activity, you will need these items:

🌶 5 or 6 child-sized knives

🌶 1 pepper or ½ pepper for each child

🌶 5 or 6 cutting boards

🌶 1 large bowl to collect the inedible parts

PROCEDURE

1. Children should wash their hands and sit at the table. When all children are sitting, teacher hands out the knives. Children use the knives safely to cut bell peppers.

2. Teacher(s) assists children as needed.

3. Teacher(s) asks children to place inedible pepper pieces in the large bowl.

4. If children are interested, have them taste the peppers and discuss texture and taste.

Remember to have children wash their hands again if they want to resume cutting peppers.

5. Clean up.

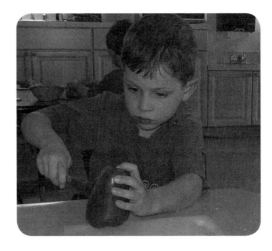

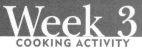

Bell Pepper Couscous Castles

ESTIMATED TIME: 35 MINUTES

RECIPE

Yields 18 servings
For this recipe, you will need these items:

FOOD INGREDIENTS

2 cups whole-wheat couscous
2 cups vegetable broth
1 cup diced bell pepper (1 large pepper)
½ cup thawed frozen corn
Nonstick cooking spray
Paprika (optional)
Ice cubes

SUPPLIES AND EQUIPMENT

Knife and cutting board for teacher
Portable large skillet
Long wooden spoons
Measuring cups and spoons
2-ounce plastic soufflé cups to use as molds
Small plates, serving tray
Plastic or flatware child-sized knives
Large mixing bowl, small bowl for ice

PROCEDURE

1. Remove the seeds and finely dice a clean bell pepper.

2. Coat a skillet well with nonstick cooking spray. Add the diced bell peppers and frozen corn to the skillet. Raise the heat to medium-high, and sauté the vegetables until tender.

3. Add the vegetable broth and couscous to the skillet. Cook, stirring constantly for about 5 minutes or until the broth has been absorbed. Remove from heat, cover, and let sit another minute or two.

4. Transfer the couscous and vegetables to a large mixing bowl and stir. While stirring, add the ice cubes one at a time, until the mixture cools enough to handle.

5. Pack the "couscous" mixture into the soufflé cups, and then turn them upside down onto the small plates to create the castles. Makes about 18 castles.

6. Transfer plates to a serving tray. If desired, lightly sprinkle with paprika. Serve individual castles and enjoy!

Suggested Ways to Involve Preschool Children in Cooking Activity:

☙ Have children wash their hands and stand or sit around the activity table. Announce, "Today we are going to make castles out of couscous and bell peppers." Ask if any children have ever heard of couscous. Explain that couscous is a tiny pasta made from wheat.

☙ To prepare the bell peppers, children can help with washing, removing seeds, and rough chopping of peppers, which you can later chop more finely with a sharp knife. To have children practice cutting, give each a plate or cutting board, a child-sized plastic knife, and a large strip of bell pepper. Invite the children to cut their strip into small pieces.

☙ Because the recipe allows the vegetables to be added to the skillet while it is still cold, invite children to scrape the diced peppers into the oiled skillet and to measure and pour in the corn.

☙ When the "couscous" mixture is cool, you can place the mixing bowl in a central location on the activity table, and the children can take the lead in making the castles. Make one as an example, and then be available to assist children as needed.

☙ As always, remember to keep children away from all sharp cutting utensils, electrical devices, and hot food and surfaces at all times!

Swiss Chard

ESTIMATED TIME: 30 MINUTES TO 1 HOUR

PURPOSE

To provide children with a beginning harvest experience as a culmination of the growing season,

- Go to the garden with a group of children and locate the Swiss chard. Discuss the planting, caring, and growing cycle as a reminder to the children.

- Demonstrate how to pick the chard and give children the opportunity to harvest the chard.

- What part of the plant are we picking? What did we do to help these chard plants grow?

To investigate Swiss chard using kitchen tools,

- Gather children inside and invite the children to help wash the chard with a salad washer.

- Provide them with child-sized kitchen scissors and bowls. Give the children opportunities to cut or tear the chard.

- What do you notice about Swiss chard?

- How is the chard the same as or different from the tomato, green beans, and bell pepper? List some ideas together.

- What are the parts of this vegetable? Can you eat all the parts? How do the different parts of the Swiss chard smell, taste, and feel?

- Introduce cutting small pieces in preparation for the cheddar and chard quesadillas.

For this activity, you will need these items:

- 5 or 6 child-sized kitchen scissors
- Several leaves of Swiss chard for each child

- 5 or 6 cutting boards
- Large bowl to collect the pieces

PROCEDURE

1. Children should wash their hands and sit at the table. When children are sitting, the teacher hands out the kitchen scissors. Children use the scissors safely to cut the chard pieces.

2. Teacher(s) assists children as needed. Children may tear the chard with their hands or cut it with scissors.

3. Teacher(s) asks children to place the chard pieces in the large bowl.

4. If children are interested, have them taste the chard and discuss texture and taste. Remember to have children wash their

hands again if they want to resume cutting chard.

5. Clean up.

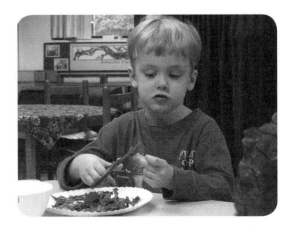

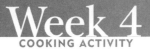

Cheddar and Chard Quesadillas
ESTIMATED TIME: 35 MINUTES

RECIPE
Yields 24 servings
For this recipe, you will need these items:

FOOD INGREDIENTS
Large bunch Swiss chard, washed, with
    stems
2 cups shredded cheddar cheese
8 whole-wheat tortillas or wraps
Canola oil
Nonstick cooking spray
Optional: salsa, low-fat sour cream,
    and/or guacamole

SUPPLIES AND EQUIPMENT
Cutting board and chef's knife for teacher
Plastic or flatware child-sized knives or
    kitchen scissors
Small plates, one per child
2 medium baking sheets
Medium saucepan
Oven, for baking
Oven mitt
Spatula, for removing quesadillas from
    baking sheets
Serving plate

PROCEDURE

1. Heat the oven to 400° F. Wash the chard and remove its stems.

2. Cut the chard into 1- to 2-inch pieces. In small amount of oil in a medium saucepan, cook the chard pieces just until tender.

3. Lightly coat the baking sheets with nonstick cooking spray.

4. Place 4 tortillas on baking sheets. Sprinkle shredded cheese evenly over the tortillas. Top the cheese with a layer of Swiss chard.

Cover the quesadillas with the remaining tortillas to create 4 quesadillas.

5. Lightly mist the tops of the quesadillas with a bit more nonstick cooking spray. Bake in the preheated oven for approximately 15 minutes.

6. Allow the quesadillas to cool. Cut each one into sixths. Transfer the pieces to a serving plate. Serve family style with low-fat sour cream, salsa, and/or guacamole, if desired. Enjoy!

Suggested Ways to Involve Preschool Children in Cooking Activity:

🌱 Have children wash their hands and sit or stand around the activity table. Announce, "Today we are going to make Cheddar and Chard Quesadillas."

🌱 Introduce all the ingredients needed for the recipe: Swiss chard, tortillas, and cheese.

🌱 Ask children to rinse the chard in the sink. Have them practice cutting the chard using child-sized knives or kitchen scissors.

🌱 Invite children to sprinkle the shredded cheese onto the tortillas. Demonstrate and then encourage them to top the cheese with a layer of chard.

🌱 Show an older child how to hold the non-stick cooking spray 6 to 8 inches away and use a gentle sweeping motion to coat the baking sheets. Younger children may then place the tortillas on the sheets.

🌱 As always, remember to keep children away from all sharp cutting utensils, electrical devices, and hot food and surfaces at all times!

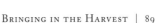

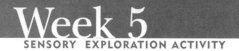

Carrots

ESTIMATED TIME: 30 MINUTES TO 1 HOUR

PURPOSE

**To provide children with a harvest experience
as a culmination of the growing season,**

- Go to the garden with a group of children and locate the carrot plants. Discuss the planting, caring, and growing cycle as a reminder to the children.

- Demonstrate how to pull the carrots and give children the opportunity to harvest them.

- What did we do to help these carrot plants to grow? What part of the plant is the part we eat?

To investigate carrots using kitchen tools,

- Gather children inside and provide them with cutting boards and child-sized knives. Remind children the carrots have been washed and cooked because it is very hard to cut raw carrots. Give the children opportunities to slice the carrots.

- What do you notice about the parts of the carrot plant?

- Where are the seeds of the carrot? Can you eat all the parts? How do the different carrot parts smell, taste, and feel? List some words to describe the carrot parts.

For this activity, you will need these items:

- 5 or 6 child-sized knives
- 2 cooked, or blanched, carrots for each child

- 5 or 6 cutting boards
- Carrots with tops
- Large bowl

Note: This sensory activity requires cooking prior to the lesson to support young children with cutting carrots. Directions: Cut carrots in half and then lengthwise. Place the pieces in a shallow pot of boiling water for 8 to 10 minutes. Cool them under cold water, and give children the cooled carrots for cutting.

PROCEDURE

1. Children should wash their hands and sit at the table. When all children are sitting, the teacher hands out the knives. Children use the knives safely to cut carrot pieces.

2. Teacher(s) assists children as needed.

3. Teacher(s) asks children to place the carrot pieces in the big bowl.

4. If children are interested, have them taste the carrots and discuss texture and taste. Remind children to wash their hands again if they want to resume cutting carrots.

5. Clean up.

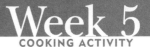
Carrot Oatmeal Cookies

ESTIMATED TIME: 20 MINUTES, PLUS 15 MINUTES BAKING TIME

RECIPE

Yields about 18 cookies

For this recipe, you will need these items:

FOOD INGREDIENTS

½ cup sugar

½ cup canola or vegetable oil

2 cups (6 ounces) shredded carrots,
    about 3 medium to large carrots

2 large eggs

2 cups white whole-wheat flour

1 cup rolled oats

1 teaspoon ground cinnamon

1 teaspoon baking powder

1½ teaspoons salt

1 teaspoon vanilla

Nonstick cooking spray

SUPPLIES AND EQUIPMENT

Food processor or hand grater

Small, medium, and large mixing bowls

Measuring cups and spoons

Fork

Mixing spoon

Large dinner spoon

2 baking sheets

Oven for baking

Oven mitt for teacher

Spatula to remove cookies from sheets

Serving plate

White whole-wheat flour is a lighter and milder type of whole-wheat flour. It is made from hard white spring wheat.

PROCEDURE

1. Heat the oven to 375° F.

2. Spray the baking sheets with nonstick cooking spray, and wash the carrots and grate them using a food processor or hand grater.

3. In a medium bowl, use a fork to beat the oil and sugar together until they're well combined.

4. In a separate small bowl, beat the two eggs using a fork. Add the beaten eggs to the oil mixture. Add the grated carrots.

5. In a large bowl, combine flour, oats,

cinnamon, baking powder, and salt. Stir until evenly combined.

6. Create a large well, or indentation, in the middle of the dry ingredients. Slowly add the oil mixture to the well. Stir until evenly combined.

7. Using a large dinner spoon, drop the batter onto a cookie sheet, leaving a 2-inch space between cookies.

8. Bake for 15 to 18 minutes or until golden brown, and allow the cookies to cool before you serve them.

Suggested Ways to Involve Preschool Children in Cooking Activity:

❧ Children wash their hands and sit or stand around the activity table. Announce, "Today we will make Carrot Oatmeal Cookies."

❧ To prepare the carrots, children can wash them. If using a hand grater, teacher can hold the grater while children grate the carrots, taking safety precautions to ensure children are not in danger of injuring their hands.

❧ Show an older child how to hold the non-stick cooking spray 6 to 8 inches away and use a gentle sweeping motion to coat the baking sheets.

❧ Children can help scoop the cookie dough and drop it onto the baking sheets.

❧ As always, remember to keep children away from all sharp cutting utensils, electrical devices, and hot food and surfaces at all times!

Butternut Squash

ESTIMATED TIME: 30 MINUTES TO 1 HOUR

PURPOSE

**To provide children with a harvest experience
as a culmination of the growing season,**

- Go to the garden with a group of children and locate the butternut squash. Discuss the planting, caring, and growing cycle as a reminder to the children.

- Demonstrate how to pick the squash and give children the opportunity to harvest the squash.

- What part of the plant are we picking? What did we do to help these squash plants grow?

To investigate butternut squash using kitchen tools,

- Gather children inside and provide them with bowls, spoons, and child-sized knives.

- Have several cooked squash available. Briefly compare the cooked and uncooked squash. Give children opportunities to cut open the squash, dig for seeds, and scoop flesh away from skin.

- What do you notice about the squash?

- How is the squash the same as or different from the tomato, green bean, bell pepper, and carrot? List some ideas together.

- What are the parts of this vegetable? Can you eat all the parts? How do the different parts of the squash smell, taste, and feel?

- Use mashers to mash the squash pieces.

For this activity, you will need these items:

- 5 or 6 child-sized knives
- 5 or 6 mashers
- 5 or 6 spoons
- 1 raw and 2 cooked squash

- 5 or 6 cutting boards
- Large bowl to collect the inedible parts
- Large bowl to collect the edible parts

Note: This sensory activity requires cooking prior to the activity. Cut squash in half lengthwise and bake in shallow dish with 1½ inches water at 350° F for 40 minutes. To avoid burning, replenish the water if it is low. Cool and give children the cooked butternut squash for mashing.

PROCEDURE

1. Children wash their hands and sit at the table. When all children are sitting, the teacher hands out the knives and spoons. Children use knives and spoons safely to cut and scoop the precooked squash.

2. Teacher(s) assists children as needed.

3. Teacher(s) asks children to place the squash pieces in the large bowls.

4. If children are interested, have them taste the squash and discuss texture and taste. Remind children to wash their hands again if they want to resume cutting the squash.

5. Clean up.

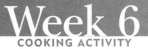

Butternut Squash Pancakes
ESTIMATED TIME: 30 MINUTES

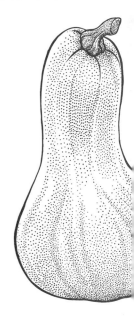

RECIPE
Yields 18 pancakes
For this recipe, you will need these items:

FOOD INGREDIENTS
1½ cups cooked butternut squash
1 cup white whole-wheat flour*
¼ teaspoon salt
1 tablespoon canola oil
1 teaspoon cinnamon
2 teaspoons baking powder
2 teaspoons brown sugar
1¼ cups milk
1 egg
Nonstick cooking spray
Maple syrup (if desired)

SUPPLIES AND EQUIPMENT
Blender
Griddle or large skillet
Cooktop or portable burner
Spoons to scoop squash
Spatula
Measuring cups and spoons

White whole-wheat flour is a lighter and milder type of whole wheat flour. It is made from hard white spring wheat.

PROCEDURE

1. Scoop cooked squash out of skin and measure out 1½ cups.

2. Combine squash, flour, cinnamon, brown sugar, salt, baking powder, canola oil, egg, and milk in the blender. Blend until well combined.

3. Lightly coat a griddle or large skillet with nonstick cooking spray.

4. Pour the batter onto the griddle into silver-dollar-sized pancakes.

5. When the batter is fairly covered with bubbles, flip the pancakes. Cook until both sides are golden brown.

6. Allow to cool slightly and, if desired, serve with warm maple syrup.

7. Enjoy!

Suggested Ways to Involve Preschool Children in Cooking Activity:

☙ Children wash their hands and sit or stand around the activity table. Announce, "Today we are going to make a recipe called Butternut Squash Pancakes."

☙ Introduce and briefly describe the origin of each ingredient for the recipe as you place it on the activity table.

☙ To prepare the squash, children can help scoop the cooled, cooked squash out of its skin.

☙ To combine ingredients, older children (four- to five-year-olds) can measure and younger children (two- to three-year-olds) can pour wet and dry ingredients into the blender.

☙ Children can take turns turning on and off the blender.

☙ As always, remember to keep children away from all sharp cutting utensils, electrical devices, and hot food and surfaces at all times!

Other Garden and Harvest Activities

Here are additional activities you can include in your classroom during these six weeks:

- Bring the inedible parts of each plant into the classroom and measure the length of vines, stems, and leaves.

- Using crayons and paper, make rubbings of the various inedible plant parts, such as the leaf (but not the chard!), stem, and vine. Then compare the rubbings.

- Using cutting tools, investigate the entire plant. Cut the stem lengthwise and discover what is inside. Use a magnifier to see the small seeds.

- Play a Garden Scavenger Hunt game. Ask, "Does anyone know the names of any of the plant's parts?" Point to each plant part—flower, fruit, leaves, stem, roots, and seeds—as the children name them.

NINE

HARVEST TIME IS COMING TO AN END
Bringing the Garden Indoors

WEEKS 7–12

THE INDOOR GARDEN ACTIVITIES encourage our child scientists to deepen their observation skills, develop comparative descriptions of the vegetables, and find special characteristics of each vegetable. The Indoor Garden Activities promote other explorations:

- Making comparisons of the vegetables through the discovery and discussion of the similarities and differences among vegetable families

- Increasing descriptive vocabulary

- Identifying vegetables by their attributes and comparing cooked and raw forms of each vegetable

Please note that when comparing vegetables, we choose not to put value on the favorite taste of a particular vegetable but encourage children to describe the characteristics of the vegetable. For instance, when comparing red, yellow, and green bell peppers, instead of saying, "Which bell pepper is your favorite?" we say, "Which one is juiciest?" "Which one is crunchiest?" "Which one is smallest?" "Which one is smoothest?" These questions increase children's vocabularies and help them to develop knowledge about the vegetable rather than making a judgment about the vegetable.

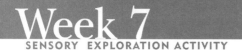

Cherry Tomatoes

ESTIMATED TIME: 30 MINUTES TO 1 HOUR

PURPOSE

To provide children with a comparison experience using cherry, grape, and plum tomatoes,

- Gather the children and identify each tomato by name. Ask children whether they have eaten fruit with these names.

- Discuss why each tomato may have been given its name.

To investigate tomatoes using kitchen tools,

- Remind children that the tomatoes have been washed—or have the children wash them. Give children opportunities to cut and scrape the tomatoes.

- What do you notice about the skin of each tomato?

- What do you notice about the inside of each tomato? How do the different parts of the tomatoes smell, taste, and feel?

Conduct a tasting investigation and record the characteristics of the tomato,

- Which tomato is juiciest?

- Which is most sour?

- Which is sweetest?

- Which is softest?

For this activity, you will need these items:

- 5 or 6 child-sized knives

- 5 or 6 cutting boards

- Cherry, grape, and plum tomatoes, enough for a group of 2 or 3 children to investigate each type

- Large bowl to collect the tomato pieces

PROCEDURE

1. Children wash their hands and sit at the table. When all children are sitting, teacher hands out the knives. Children use knives safely to cut tomato pieces.

2. Teacher(s) assists children as needed.

3. Teacher(s) asks children to place the tomato pieces in the big bowl.

4. If children are interested, have them taste the tomatoes and discuss texture and taste. Record the tomatoes' characteristics. Remind children to wash their hands again if they want to resume cutting tomatoes.

5. Clean up.

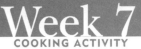

Pasta with Garlic-Parmesan Tomato Sauce

ESTIMATED TIME: 25 MINUTES

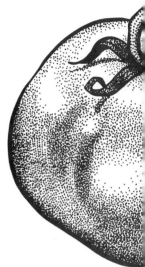

RECIPE

Yields 18 servings
For this recipe, you will need these items:

FOOD INGREDIENTS

½ pound whole-wheat pasta
2 quarts water for boiling pasta
3 cloves fresh garlic—2 to cook with plus
   1 to pass around
3 cups cherry tomatoes, washed
2 tablespoons olive oil
¼ cup vegetable or low-sodium chicken
   broth, or bouillon cubes dissolved in
   ¼ cup of water
4 heaping tablespoons grated Parmesan
   cheese

SUPPLIES AND EQUIPMENT

Chef's knife, cutting board for teacher
Handheld garlic press
Measuring spoons and cups
Blender or food processor
Large pasta pot, colander
Large skillet with heat source
Long wooden spoon
Small plates, one per child, plus extra
Plastic or flatware child-sized knives
Timer
Serving dish and large spoon

PROCEDURE

1. In the large pasta pot, bring approximately 2 quarts of water to a rolling boil on high heat.

2. Meanwhile, rinse any unwashed cherry tomatoes. Cut all of the tomatoes in half.

3. After removing the outer skin, crush the garlic in the press and set it aside.

4. Add 1 tablespoon olive oil to the water to help prevent the noodles from sticking together. Then add the pasta and cook for approximately 10 minutes (or as directed on the package).

5. Add the halved tomatoes and broth to the blender or food processor. Use the pulse mechanism on the blender to coarsely chop and incorporate the ingredients.

6. When the pasta has finished cooking, remove it from the heat, drain it, and rinse with cold water to stop it from cooking.

7. Heat the remaining olive oil in the skillet on medium-high heat. When the oil is hot, add about 2 teaspoons of the crushed garlic and cook for 30 seconds. Then add the blended tomato sauce from the blender. Reduce heat and simmer for about 5 minutes to cook off excess liquid and concentrate the flavor.

8. Add the cooked pasta to the skillet and stir to coat it with the sauce. Heat for another minute or two. Then remove from heat and transfer to a serving dish.

9. Stir 3 heaping tablespoons of the grated Parmesan cheese into the hot pasta dish. Sprinkle the remaining cheese on top. Serve family style and enjoy!

Suggested Ways to Involve Preschool Children in Cooking Activity:

☀ Children wash their hands and sit or stand around the activity table.

☀ Pass around a piece of uncooked pasta and talk about its shape. Tell the children that the pasta comes from wheat grains that have been ground into flour.

☀ Cheese, please! Children may carry out the steps of adding the grated Parmesan cheese at the end of the recipe.

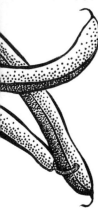

Green Beans

ESTIMATED TIME: 30 MINUTES TO 1 HOUR

PURPOSE

To support children in naming the target vegetables,

❦ Ask children to name each of the target vegetables. You may need to give clues by describing color, size, or shape.

To prompt children to identify green beans through a tactile experience,

❦ Pass around a mystery bag so each child has a turn to put a hand in to feel the vegetable. Remind children to wait for everyone to have a turn. What words can they use to describe what they have felt? Ask children the name of the vegetable.

To develop fine-motor skills by investigating the green beans using kitchen tools,

❦ Have children use child-sized kitchen scissors to explore the insides of the green bean.

For this activity, you will need these items:

❦ 5 or 6 child-sized kitchen scissors

❦ 2 or 3 green beans per child

❦ 5 or 6 cutting boards

❦ 1 large bowl to collect the bean pieces

❦ 1 mystery bag (a small paper bag or drawstring cloth bag used to hide the green bean)

PROCEDURE

1. Children wash their hands and sit at the activity table. Challenge children to name each target vegetable. Assist children by providing some words that describe each vegetable.

2. Pass around the mystery bag with a green bean inside. Give each child a turn to reach in and touch the vegetable. Ask each child to wait quietly until everyone has had a turn. (You might want to have several bags so a number of children can reach into mystery bags at the same time because it's hard for them to wait quietly in a group larger than three or four.) Ask each child to describe what is in the bag and perhaps name the object. Listen to their guesses and consider the possibilities. When each child has had a turn, the teacher will slowly reach in the bag and pull out the green bean (typically to cheering children)!

3. Pass out 2 or 3 beans per child and one pair of child-sized kitchen scissors. Have children cut small pieces. Children can count their pieces, measure and compare their pieces, and taste their pieces. Remind children to wash their hands again if they want to resume cutting beans.

4. Ask children to place bean pieces in the large bowl when they're done investigating.

5. Clean up.

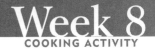

Green Bean Wontons with Dipping Sauce

ESTIMATED TIME: 40 MINUTES

RECIPE
Yields 40 wontons
For this recipe, you will need these items:

FOOD INGREDIENTS
3 cups shredded green beans (1 pound)
40 wonton wrappers
2 tablespoons canola oil
4 tablespoons rice vinegar
2 tablespoons low-sodium tamari
   (wheat-free soy sauce)
2 teaspoons honey

SUPPLIES AND EQUIPMENT
Nonstick skillet and heat source
Spatula, small ladle
Measuring spoons and cups
Mixing spoon, medium bowl
Small bowl or cup with water
Paper bowls, one per child, plus extra
Small plates, one per child, plus extra
Food processor

PROCEDURE

1. Clean and remove the stems from green beans. Shred the green beans in a food processor. Set the shredded green beans aside.

2. Heat the oil in a nonstick skillet over medium to high heat. Sauté the shredded green beans until they're tender.

3. To create a green bean wonton, take one wonton wrapper, place ½ tablespoon of shredded green beans in the center of the wrapper, wet all sides of the wonton with your finger, and fold the wonton to form a triangle. Press the edges together. Repeat until you've made the desired number of wontons.

4. Heat a small amount of oil in the nonstick skillet.

5. Sauté the wontons 2 to 3 minutes per side or until slightly golden.

6. While the wontons are cooking, prepare the dipping sauce by mixing tamari, rice vinegar, and honey in a small bowl.

7. Remove the wontons from the skillet and serve with the dipping sauce as soon as they are cool enough to eat safely.

Suggested Ways to Involve Preschool Children in Cooking Activity:

🖑 Children wash their hands and sit or stand around the activity table. Announce, "Today we will make a recipe called Green Bean Wontons. We'll use green beans like the ones we grew in our garden."

🖑 Introduce and briefly describe the origin of each ingredient for the recipe as you place it on the activity table. For example, you can explain that the word *tamari* means liquid pressed from soybeans and that the sauce originated in China.

🖑 To prepare the green beans, children can help wash them and remove their stems.

🖑 Children may enjoy watching you process the green beans.

🖑 To combine the dipping ingredients, older children (four- to five-year-olds) can measure and younger children (two- to three-year-olds) can pour the ingredients into the mixing bowl. One child can stir with the mixing spoon while others hold the bowl steady.

🖑 Children enjoy filling and folding their own wontons.

🖑 As always, remember to keep children away from all sharp cutting utensils, electrical devices, and hot food and surfaces at all times!

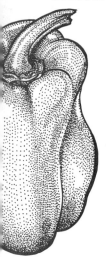

Bell Peppers

ESTIMATED TIME: 30 MINUTES TO 1 HOUR

PURPOSE

To compare red, yellow, and green bell peppers,

❦ Have a discussion about how whole bell peppers are different from and similar to each other. How are the peppers the same? How are the peppers different?

❦ Give each child a piece of the bell pepper with skin, flesh, and seeds. Ask the child to describe what she sees and feels. Ask all of the children to discard the seeds and cut peppers for tasting when they are done investigating.

To conduct a tasting activity and record the results,

❦ Provide children with the opportunity to taste each bell pepper and record their descriptions. Which bell pepper is the juiciest? Which is the crunchiest? Which is the sweetest?

For this activity, you will need these items:

❦ 6 bell peppers (2 each of red, green, and yellow)

❦ 1 adult knife for the teacher

❦ 5 small bowls

❦ 5 child-sized knives

❦ 1 storage tray

❦ Large bowl for discarding inedible parts

PROCEDURE

1. Children wash their hands and sit or stand at the activity table.

2. Children describe similarities and differences of the bell peppers.

3. Teacher hands out the knives. Children use knives to carefully cut the peppers and describe what they notice on the inside. Identify the various parts. Where is the skin? Where are the seeds?

4. Teacher(s) assists children as needed.

5. Teacher(s) asks children to place pepper pieces in the large bowl.

6. Conduct a taste investigation of each pepper and support children in describing the pepper's characteristics. Record the results. Remember to have children wash their hands again if they want to resume cutting bell peppers.

7. Clean up.

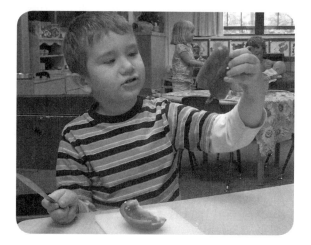

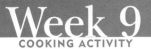

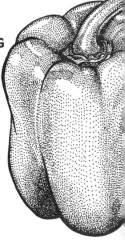

Confetti Corn Muffins

ESTIMATED TIME: 20 MINUTES, PLUS 30 MINUTES FOR BAKING AND COOLING

RECIPE
Yields 18 mini muffins
For this recipe, you will need these items:

FOOD INGREDIENTS
1 cup cornmeal (fine milled)
½ cup white whole-wheat flour
¼ teaspoon salt
1 teaspoon baking powder
½ teaspoon baking soda
1½ cups low-fat plain yogurt
3 tablespoons honey
2 large eggs
3 tablespoons canola or safflower oil
½ bell pepper, any color
¾ cup shredded sharp cheddar cheese
Nonstick cooking spray

SUPPLIES AND EQUIPMENT
Large and medium mixing bowls
Measuring spoons and cups
Long wooden spoon
Wire whisk
Mini muffin baking pans, for 18 muffins
Plastic flatware child-sized knives, one
    per child
Small plates, one per child, plus extra
Chef's knife, cutting board for teacher
Small ladle, preferably 1-ounce in size
Oven and oven mitt
Basket, lined with clean towel, for serving

PROCEDURE

1. Heat the oven to 400° F. Coat muffin tins well with nonstick cooking spray.

2. Clean bell peppers and remove their seeds. Finely dice the peppers and set them aside.

3. Combine in a large mixing bowl the cornmeal, flour, salt, baking powder, and baking soda.

4. Whisk together in a medium mixing bowl the yogurt, honey, eggs, and oil.

5. Create a well, or indentation, in the center of the dry ingredient mixture and fill it with the wet mixture. Gently stir the batter until all the dry ingredients are incorporated. Do not overstir.

6. Gently fold ½ cup of shredded cheddar cheese into the batter.

7. Use a 1-ounce ladle to fill each oiled muffin cup about three-quarters full. Sprinkle the diced bell peppers on the tops of the uncooked muffins. Do the same with the remaining ¼ cup of cheddar cheese.

8. Bake 15 to 20 minutes or until the muffins are golden brown. Allow the muffins to cool slightly before you remove them from the pans. Transfer the cool muffins to lined basket. Serve family style and enjoy!

Suggested Ways to Involve Preschool Children in Cooking Activity:

❦ Children wash their hands and sit or stand around the activity table. Announce, "Today we are going to make a recipe called Confetti Corn Muffins."

❦ Introduce and briefly describe the origin of each ingredient for the recipe as you place it on the activity table. For example, explain that cornmeal is made from corn kernels that have been ground or crushed in a mill.

❦ To prepare the bell peppers, children can help with washing, removing seeds, and rough chopping of peppers, which you can finely chop with a sharp knife later.

❦ Children enjoy sprinkling the shredded cheese and bell pepper pieces on top of the muffins before baking.

Swiss Chard

ESTIMATED TIME: 30 MINUTES TO 1 HOUR

PURPOSE
**To help children compare three different
green leafy vegetables in cooked and raw form,**

- We grew a green leafy vegetable in our garden. Do you know its name?

- Today we will explore and compare three green leafy vegetables. Ask children to try to name the vegetables.

- Today we'll use our kitchen scissors or our hands to cut or tear the leaves of these vegetables. What do you notice about the inside of the leaves? What do they taste like? What words could you use to describe the taste and feel of the green leafy vegetables?

- Provide cooked and raw green leafy vegetables. Compare the textures and tastes.

For this activity, you will need these items:

- 5 or 6 child-sized kitchen scissors

- ½ bunch each of chard, collard greens, and kale (provide some cooked and raw of each)

- 5 or 6 cutting boards or plates

- Large bowl to collect the inedible greens pieces

- 1 plastic bag for storage of extra chard (to be used by teacher)

Note: This sensory activity requires cooking prior to the lesson. Sauté half the amount of each leafy green vegetable in 2 teaspoons of olive oil at medium heat for 3 minutes. Cool and give children the cooked Swiss chard for exploring.

PROCEDURE

1. Children wash their hands and sit at the activity table. When all children are sitting, the teacher hands out the kitchen scissors. Children use scissors safely to cut greens into pieces. Offer one type of green at a time and discuss the sensory experiences.

2. Teacher(s) assists children as needed and gives children the choice of using their hands for tearing or the kitchen scissors for cutting.

3. Teacher(s) asks children to compare the cooked and raw green leafy vegetables.

4. If children are interested, let them taste the greens and discuss the textures and tastes. Remind children to wash their hands again if they want to resume cutting or tearing the vegetables.

5. Clean up.

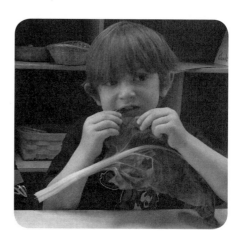

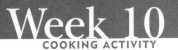
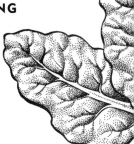

Pita Pocket Pizzas

ESTIMATED TIME: 20 MINUTES, PLUS 15 MINUTES FOR BAKING AND COOLING

RECIPE
Yields 32 pita pocket pizza slices
For this recipe you will need these items:

FOOD INGREDIENTS
1 bunch Swiss chard, washed and dried
2 tablespoons olive oil
2 cans (8 ounces) tomato sauce
½ teaspoon garlic powder
½ teaspoon Italian spices (no salt added)
1½ cups shredded mozzarella cheese
8 large whole-wheat pita bread rounds

SUPPLIES AND EQUIPMENT
Small plates, one per child
Plastic or flatware child-sized knives
Chef's knife and cutting board
Large spoon for cooking
Measuring cups and spoons
2 large bowls
Large skillet and heat source
Large baking sheet(s)

PROCEDURE

1. Heat the oven to 400° F.

2. Lay the washed chard leaves on top of one another with all stems facing the same direction. With the chef's knife, cut a triangle shape around the stems to separate all the leaves from all the stems at one time. Then stack the leaves and chop them finely.

3. Heat the oil in skillet for about 1 minute. Then add chard and cook, stirring occasionally, for 2 minutes.

4. Remove the skillet from the heat and carefully add the tomato sauce, stirring gently until the leaves and sauce are combined.

5. Add the garlic powder and spices and stir.

6. Lay out the pita bread on large baking sheet(s).

7. Spread approximately 2 tablespoons of sauce on each pita round. Sprinkle cheese on top of the sauce on each pita.

8. Bake the pita pocket pizzas for 7 to 10 minutes or until the cheese is bubbly.

9. Remove the pita pocket pizzas from oven. Cut each pita round into 4 slices, so you'll have about 2 slices per child.

10. Serve family style and enjoy!

Suggested Ways to Involve Preschool Children in Cooking Activity:

1. Children wash their hands and sit or stand around the activity table. Announce, "Today we are going to make a recipe called Pita Pocket Pizzas using chard like we grew in our garden."

2. Children of all ages can help tear chard leaves into very small pieces and place them into a large bowl, ready for you to finely chop.

3. Prior to cooking, invite each child to keep a small piece of leaf and stem to taste. Ask children to describe the chard and its taste.

4. Older children can take turns measuring the sauce and younger children can lay the pita bread on baking sheets.

5. Children can spread the sauce on the pita bread and then sprinkle the cheese on top.

6. As always, remember to keep children away from all sharp cutting utensils, electrical devices, and hot food and surfaces at all times!

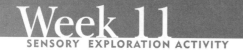

Carrots

ESTIMATED TIME: 30 MINUTES TO 1 HOUR

PURPOSE

To compare shredded cooked carrots with uncooked carrots,

☀ What do you notice about the cooked and uncooked carrots? What words could you use to describe the two kinds of carrots?

To compare baby carrots with mature carrots, focusing on taste,

☀ How are these two carrots the same/different?

☀ Describe how baby carrots are produced.

For this activity, you will need these items:

☀ 1 adult-sized grater

☀ 1 adult knife

☀ 4 to 5 potato mashers

☀ 5 child-sized bowls

☀ 5 child-sized knives

☀ 1 bowl of 2 to 3 grated, cooked carrots (prepared ahead of activity)

☀ 2 to 3 raw carrots or 1 bowl of grated raw carrots

☀ 2 to 3 raw baby carrots

Note: This sensory activity requires cooking prior to the lesson. Place grated raw carrots in a shallow pot of boiling water and cook for 5 minutes or until tender. Cool and give children the cooked carrots for mashing.

PROCEDURE

1. Children wash their hands and sit at the activity table. When all children are sitting, the teacher hands out the knives.

2. Children cut tops off carrots if they can; otherwise, teacher cuts off tops. The carrots should be cut about one-half inch from the top to include the carrot greens.

3. On the soaked paper towel on the pie plate, children arrange the carrot tops and then set the pie plate aside to observe the growth of carrot greens. Water needs to be visible in the pan and the paper towel kept soaking wet for the tops to continue to grow or stay fresh. Remember to check regularly to avoid mold. Chart the carrot tops' growth.

4. One child at a time grates a long carrot while teacher holds the grater and takes safety precautions to the ensure child does not injure fingers. Or teacher can grate the carrots ahead of time.

5. Several children mash the cooked, shredded carrots.

6. Taste the baby carrots and compare them to the cooked and raw grated carrots. Encourage children to use descriptive words for each type of carrot. Remind children to wash their hands again if they want to resume grating carrots.

7. Clean up.

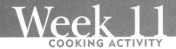

Honey Glazed Carrots

ESTIMATED TIME: 40 TO 45 MINUTES

RECIPE

Yields about 18 servings
For this recipe, you will need these items:

FOOD INGREDIENTS

12 to 15 carrots
1 tablespoon low-sodium tamari (wheat-
  free soy sauce)
2 tablespoons butter
3 tablespoons honey

SUPPLIES AND EQUIPMENT

Saucepan
Vegetable peeler
Vegetable steamer
Strainer
Measuring spoons
Wooden spoon
Knife and cutting board for teacher
Plastic child-sized knives, one per child
Small plates or cutting boards

PROCEDURE

1. Wash and peel the carrots.

2. Steam carrots until they're just tender. Rinse in a strainer under cold water to cool.

3. Cut the cooled carrots into bite-sized pieces.

4. Place the butter and tamari in the saucepan and cook over medium-low heat.

5. When the butter is melted, add the honey.

6. Stir in the steamed carrots and mix until all carrots are coated or glazed with the honey butter.

Suggested Ways to Involve Preschool Children in Cooking Activity:

❦ Children wash their hands and sit or stand around the activity table. Announce, "Today we are going to make a recipe called Honey Glazed Carrots using carrots like the ones from our garden."

❦ Introduce each ingredient as you place it on the activity table.

❦ To prepare the carrots, children can wash them. When the carrots have been steamed and cooled, encourage children to cut each carrot into bite-sized pieces using their child-sized knives.

❦ To combine ingredients, older children (four- to five-year-olds) can measure and younger children (two- to three-year-olds) can pour ingredients into the skillet.

❦ As always, remember to keep children away from all sharp cutting utensils, electrical devices, and hot food and surfaces at all times!

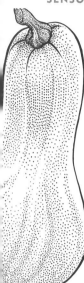

Butternut Squash
ESTIMATED TIME: 30 MINUTES TO 1 HOUR

PURPOSE
Compare cooked butternut squash with spaghetti squash,

🌱 What do you notice about the spaghetti squash and butternut squash?

🌱 What words could you use to describe the two kinds of squash?

For this activity, you will need these items:

🌱 ½ raw butternut squash

🌱 ½ raw spaghetti squash

🌱 ½ cooked butternut squash

🌱 ½ cooked spaghetti squash

🌱 4 to 5 potato mashers

🌱 5 child-sized bowls

🌱 5 child-sized knives

🌱 1 storage tray

🌱 Large bowl to collect pieces

Note: This sensory activity requires cooking prior to the activity. Cut squash in half lengthwise and bake in shallow dish with 1½ inches water at 350° F for 40 minutes. To avoid burning, replenish the water if it is low. Remove seeds and cool. Give the children the cooled butternut squash for comparing.

PROCEDURE

1. Children wash their hands and sit at the activity table.

2. The teacher introduces the two types of squash to children by showing the two uncooked squashes. Compare the color and texture of the skin.

3. Provide children with pieces of squash that have been cooked, cooled, and seeds removed. Children can use knives and mashers to investigate the consistency of the squash and share descriptions of the process.

4. If children are interested, they can taste the spaghetti and butternut squash and compare the two. Describe the taste, texture, and color of each squash. Remind children to wash their hands again if they want to resume cutting squash.

5. Clean up.

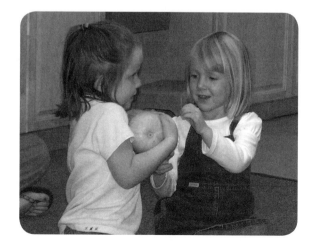

Banana Squash Smoothie
ESTIMATED TIME: 20 MINUTES

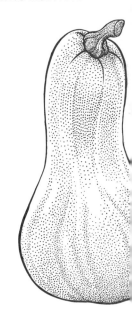

RECIPE
Yields about 18 servings
For this recipe, you will need these items:

FOOD INGREDIENTS

1½ cups butternut squash (cut in half lengthwise, baked, seeds left intact)
3 cups low-fat milk
1½ cups low-fat vanilla yogurt
1½ ripe bananas
1½ teaspoons vanilla

SUPPLIES AND EQUIPMENT

Blender, oven
Small cups (3- to 5-ounce size)
Large bowl for scooped squash
Medium bowl for seeds
Measuring cups and spoons
Spoons

PROCEDURE

1. Cut squash in half lengthwise, leaving seeds intact, and bake until tender.

2. Scoop seeds out of squash and discard.

3. Scoop squash out of skin and measure 1½ cups of it.

4. Combine in blender squash, milk, banana, vanilla, and yogurt.

5. Blend very well until smooth.

Suggested Ways to Involve Preschool Children in Cooking Activity:

- Announce, "Today we are going to make a recipe called Banana Squash Smoothies using butternut squash like we grew in our garden."

- Introduce each ingredient for the recipe as you place it on the activity table: cooked butternut squash, milk, banana, and vanilla yogurt. Place the blender in a central location on the table or counter used for activity.

- Children can help remove seeds from the squash by gently scraping the seeds out with spoons. They can also help peel the banana.

- Have children take turns measuring the ingredients into the unplugged blender or into a separate container.

- Plug in the blender and move children away from the electric cord. It may be fun for children to push the buttons on the blender!

- Please remember to keep electric cords and blender blades away from the reach of children.

Other Activities to Bring the Garden Indoors

Here are additional activities you can include in your classroom during these six weeks:

- Create a mystery bag (a drawstring cloth bag). Put three long, thin green vegetables, such as a celery stalk, a green bean, and a pepper slice, in the bag. Ask children to choose the green bean.

- Compare yellow and green beans. Ask if the colors, textures, and tastes are the same or different.

- Compare cooked carrots and uncooked carrots. Taste uncooked and cooked carrot slices and ask questions about the texture and taste.

- Compare various winter squashes, such as delicata, acorn, and pumpkin, to butternut squash. Ask questions about the similarities and differences of the seeds, flesh, taste, and texture of each squash.

⤳ TEN ⤝

PUTTING THE GARDEN TO SLEEP
Indoor Winter Activities

WEEKS 13–18

THE WINTER CURRICULUM ENCOURAGES CHILDREN and adults to work at a slower pace and to try food preparation methods of the past, such as canning, drying, and using handheld tools when cooking. The activities in this section promote:

- The historical perspective of food, such as drying vegetables
- Developing fine-motor skills through the use of kitchen tools
- Comparing handheld kitchen tools with modern appliances
- Exploring cooked and uncooked target vegetables
- Providing a model of adult work and of slowing down to assist in the understanding of the seed-to-table experience

Tomatoes

ESTIMATED TIME: 30 MINUTES TO 1 HOUR

PURPOSE
To provide children with winter uses of tomatoes,

🌱 Gather children and review the tomato with them. Using a photo of tomatoes, ask children what they remember from growing and harvesting the tomatoes.

🌱 Explain the necessity of drying vegetables and how to use dried vegetables all winter long.

🌱 Provide children with cherry tomatoes, cutting boards, and child-sized knives. Remind children to use the knives safely as they cut the tomatoes into halves.

🌱 Ask children what will happen when they dry the tomatoes. What will happen to the juice? What will happen to the seeds?

For this activity, you will need these items:

🌱 Photo of tomatoes

🌱 5 or 6 child-sized knives

🌱 2 or 3 cherry tomatoes per child

🌱 5 or 6 cutting boards

🌱 Baking sheet with parchment paper

🌱 Dehydrator or oven for drying

PROCEDURE

1. Heat the oven to 140° F.

2. Children wash their hands and sit at the activity table. When all children are sitting, the teacher hands out the knives. Children use knives safely to cut cherry tomatoes into halves.

3. Teacher(s) assists children as needed.

4. Teacher(s) asks children to place the tomato pieces on the baking sheet.

5. If children are interested, let them taste the tomatoes and discuss what the taste might be like when the tomatoes are dried.

6. Remind children to wash their hands again if they want to resume cutting tomatoes.

7. After the tomatoes are placed on baking sheet, have an adult put the sheet in the preheated oven and dry the tomatoes for 4 to 8 hours. Or use a dehydrator set between 135° F and 140° F. Space the tomatoes 1 inch apart and dry them for 9 to 12 hours or until dried.

8. Clean up.

9. When the tomatoes have dried, invite children to sample the dehydrated tomatoes.

Note: Drying is an ancient form of food preservation that removes water from the food.

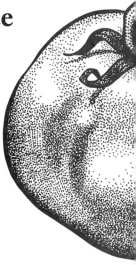

English Muffin Pizzas with Homemade Sauce
ESTIMATED TIME: 20 MINUTES, PLUS 15 MINUTES BAKING TIME

RECIPE
Yields 16 to 32 slices
For this recipe, you will need these items:

FOOD INGREDIENTS
2 cups cherry tomatoes, washed (about 20 tomatoes)
1 tablespoon olive oil
1 teaspoon sugar
4 whole-wheat English muffins
1½ cups shredded, part-skim mozzarella cheese

SUPPLIES AND EQUIPMENT
Plastic or flatware child-sized knives
Chef's knife, cutting board for teacher
Blender or food processor
Medium baking sheet
Colander, for washing tomatoes
Large skillet with heat source
Wooden spoon for sautéing
Small plates
Measuring cups and spoons
Small, shallow bowl, serving platter
Spoon for spreading sauce
Oven for baking, oven mitt
Spatula for removing pizzas

PROCEDURE

1. Heat oven to 400° F. Rinse the cherry tomatoes.

2. Children may halve cherry tomatoes.

3. Heat 1 tablespoon olive oil in the skillet over medium heat. Add the halved tomatoes to the skillet and sprinkle them with sugar. Sauté for 5 to 6 minutes.

4. Transfer the skillet's contents to a blender or food processor and purée the mixture. Pour the purée into a shallow bowl.

5. Split the English muffins in half and place the halves on ungreased baking sheet.

6. To assemble each pizza, spoon about 2 tablespoons of sauce onto English muffin "crusts." Use the back of the spoon to spread the sauce. Cover the sauce with a handful of cheese.

7. Bake the pizzas in the oven for 10 to 15 minutes or until the cheese is bubbly and just beginning to brown.

8. Allow the pizzas to cool slightly and cut them in halves or quarters. Transfer the slices to a serving platter, serve family style, and enjoy!

Suggested Ways to Involve Preschool Children in Cooking Activity:

☙ Children wash their hands and sit or stand around the cooking activity table. Announce, "Today we are going to make English Muffin Pizzas with Homemade Sauce using cherry tomatoes."

☙ Children can rinse the cherry tomatoes. They can practice cutting the tomatoes in half on plates, using the child-sized knives.

☙ Each child can assemble one English muffin pizza. Pass the bowl of sauce, followed by the bowl of cheese, around the activity table. Assist as needed.

☙ As always, remember to keep children away from all sharp cutting utensils, electrical devices, and hot food and surfaces at all times!

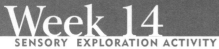

Green Beans

ESTIMATED TIME: 30 MINUTES TO 1 HOUR

PURPOSE
**To provide children with the experience of cooked and raw beans
and to offer the history of the green bean,**

- Gather children and review the green bean. Using a photo of green beans, ask children if they remember how the plant grew in the garden. What color were the beans from the garden? Why are green beans called *string beans*?

- Provide children with green beans, cutting boards, and child-sized knives. Remind children to use knives safely when they cut the cooked and raw beans. Guide children to describe the inside of each bean pod. Do they have to peel a string to get inside?

- Ask children to describe the cooked and raw green beans. Which is easier to cut? Which is the juiciest? Which is the crunchiest? How are they the same? How are they different?

For this activity, you will need these items:

- Photo of green beans

- 5 or 6 child-sized knives

- 4 green beans per child (2 cooked, 2 raw)

- 5 or 6 cutting boards

- Large bowl to collect cut green beans

Note: This sensory activity requires cooking prior to the lesson. Place washed, cut green beans in a shallow pan of boiling water. Cook the beans for 5 to 8 minutes or until tender. Cool the beans before use with the children.

PROCEDURE

1. Children wash their hands and sit at the activity table. When all children are sitting, teacher hands out the knives. Children use knives safely to cut green bean pieces.

2. Teacher(s) assists children as needed.

3. Teacher(s) asks children guiding questions.

4. If children are interested, let them taste the green beans and discuss texture and taste. Remind children to wash their hands again if they want to resume cutting green beans.

5. Clean up.

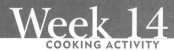
Sesame Seed Green Beans

ESTIMATED TIME: 30 MINUTES

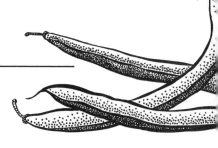

RECIPE

Yields about 18 servings
For this recipe, you will need these items:

FOOD INGREDIENTS

1 to 1½ pounds fresh green beans
1 tablespoon olive oil
Salt and pepper to taste
½ cup sesame seeds in a shaker

SUPPLIES AND EQUIPMENT

Large skillet
Measuring spoon
Long wooden spoon
Plastic or flatware child-sized knives

PROCEDURE

1. Wash and trim the ends from green beans. Snap the beans in half.

2. Pour the oil into a skillet and warm it over medium heat.

3. Add the green beans to the skillet and sauté the beans until they're tender.

4. Season the beans with salt and pepper.

5. Serve the beans in small bowls and enjoy! Invite children to sprinkle sesame seeds on their green beans if they like.

Suggested Ways to Involve Preschool Children in Cooking Activity:

❦ Children wash their hands and sit or stand around the activity table. Announce, "Today we are going to make a recipe called Sesame Seed Green Beans."

❦ Introduce and briefly describe the origin of each ingredient for the recipe as you place it on the activity table.

❦ To prepare the green beans, children can wash the beans, snap off their stems, and snap the beans in half.

❦ Children can season cooked beans with salt and pepper and sprinkle sesame seeds on their beans if they choose.

❦ As always, remember to keep children away from all sharp cutting utensils, electrical devices, and hot food and surfaces at all times!

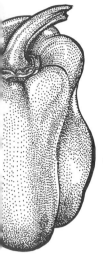

Bell Peppers

ESTIMATED TIME: 30 MINUTES TO 1 HOUR

PURPOSE

To provide children with the experience of exploring the bell pepper in cooked and raw form and using knives to dice bell peppers,

❧ Gather children and review the bell pepper. Using a photo of bell peppers, ask children if they remember how the plant grew in the garden. What color were the bell peppers from the garden? What color peppers have the children tried?

❧ Provide each child with half a bell pepper, cutting board, and child-sized plastic knife. Remind children to use knives safely as they cut the bell peppers. Guide children to describe the inside of each bell pepper. Use knives to dice the peppers (that is, cut them into very small pieces).

❧ Ask children to describe the cooked and raw pepper. Which is easier to cut? Which is crunchiest? Which is juiciest? How are the peppers similar? How are the peppers different?

For this activity, you will need these items:

❧ Photo of bell peppers

❧ 5 or 6 child-sized knives

❧ ½ pepper per child (¼ cooked and ¼ raw)

❧ 5 or 6 cutting boards

❧ Large bowl to collect cuttings and seeds

Note: This sensory activity requires cooking prior to the lesson. Spray a cooking sheet evenly with nonstick cooking spray. Place cut raw bell peppers on the cooking sheet and bake at 350° F for 10 minutes. Provide the children with the cooled bell peppers for exploration.

PROCEDURE

1. Children wash their hands and sit at the activity table. When all children are sitting, teacher hands out the knives. Children use knives safely to cut bell pepper pieces.

2. Teacher(s) assists children as needed.

3. Teacher(s) asks children guiding questions. Talk with children about cutting, or dicing, the bell pepper in very small pieces. Compare the cooked pepper with the raw pepper.

4. If children are interested, let them taste the bell peppers and discuss texture and taste.

   Remind children to wash their hands again if they want to resume cutting bell peppers.

5. Clean up.

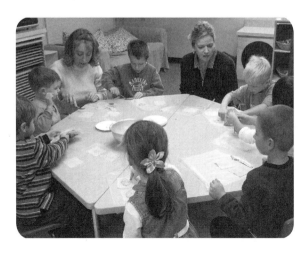

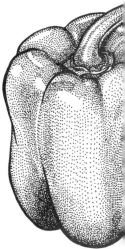

Bell Pepper Veggie Burgers
ESTIMATED TIME: 35 MINUTES

RECIPE
Yields 18 small patties
For this recipe, you will need these items:

FOOD INGREDIENTS
22 ounces (1½ 15-ounce cans) canned
   black beans
1 cup Italian bread crumbs
1 large red bell pepper
3 eggs
2 teaspoons vegetable oil
¾ cup shredded cheddar cheese
8 small or 4 large whole-wheat pita
   pockets
Nonstick cooking spray
Ketchup for serving

SUPPLIES AND EQUIPMENT
Manual can opener, large baking sheet
Large mixing bowl, strainer
Chef's knife, cutting board for teacher
Long wooden spoon, dry measuring cups
Small bowl for beating eggs
Whisk or fork for beating eggs
Potato masher or large fork
Skillet with heat source
Small plates, one per child
Plastic or flatware child-sized knives
Spatula for removing burgers from pan
Oven for broiling, oven mitt

PROCEDURE

1. Heat the oven to broil.* Spray the baking sheet generously with nonstick cooking spray.

2. Wash the bell pepper and remove its stem and seeds. Cut the pepper into small pieces.

3. Place the vegetable oil in a skillet. Heat the oil over medium heat and add the pepper pieces. Sauté the pepper pieces until they are tender.

4. In a small bowl, lightly beat the eggs with a fork or whisk.

5. Drain the canned beans, and rinse the beans with cool water. Place the beans in a large bowl and mash them well using a potato masher or large fork.

6. Add and stir until evenly combined: peppers, bread crumbs, lightly beaten eggs, and cheese.

7. Form the burger mixture into 18 small patties and place them on the baking sheet. Place in oven 4 to 6 inches below broiler flame. Broil the burgers for 5 minutes, flip them, and broil them an additional 5 to 6 minutes. Watch closely to prevent burning.

8. When the burgers are done, allow them to cool slightly before you place them in halved or quartered pita pockets. Serve them with plenty of ketchup and enjoy!

* Burgers can also be cooked on the stovetop in a skillet coated with a small amount of vegetable oil. Cook over medium-high heat for 4 to 5 minutes on each side.

Suggested Ways to Involve Preschool Children in Cooking Activity:

☙ Children wash their hands and sit or stand around the cooking activity table. Announce, "Today we are going to make Bell Pepper Veggie Burgers using red bell peppers."

☙ Introduce all of the ingredients needed to make the burgers: beans, bell peppers, bread crumbs, eggs, cheese, pita bread, and ketchup.

☙ Children can rinse the bell pepper and remove its seeds. Invite children to sample a small piece of the bell pepper.

☙ Show children how to form the burger mixture into small patties and place them on the baking sheet. Remind children to wash their hands again after they have handled the burger mixture.

Swiss Chard

ESTIMATED TIME: 30 MINUTES TO 1 HOUR

PURPOSE
To provide children with the experience
of exploring Swiss chard in cooked and raw forms,

🌱 Gather children and review the Swiss chard. Using a photo of chard, ask children if they remember how the plant grew in the garden. What color were the leaves and stems?

🌱 Provide children with chard leaves, cutting boards, and child-sized kitchen scissors. Remind children to use the scissors safely as they cut the chard. Guide children to describe the parts of the chard leaves and stems.

🌱 Ask children their preference. Which is easier to cut? Which is the smoothest? Which is crunchiest? How are the cooked and raw Swiss chard similar? How are they different?

For this activity, you will need these items:

🌱 Photo of Swiss chard

🌱 5 or 6 child-sized kitchen scissors

🌱 2 chard leaves per child (1 cooked, 1 raw)

🌱 5 or 6 cutting boards

🌱 Large bowl to collect pieces

Note: This sensory activity requires cooking prior to the lesson. Separate half of the raw chard and place 5 or 6 leaves of the chard in 2 teaspoons of heated olive oil and sauté for 3 minutes. Repeat until you have cooked enough for each child to have one cooked leaf. Provide children with the chard after it has cooled.

PROCEDURE

1. Children wash their hands and sit at the activity table. When all children are sitting, the teacher hands out the kitchen scissors. Children use the scissors safely to cut chard pieces.

2. Teacher(s) assists children as needed.

3. Teacher(s) asks children guiding questions.

4. If children are interested, let them taste the chard and discuss texture and taste. Remind children to wash their hands again if they want to resume cutting chard.

5. Clean up.

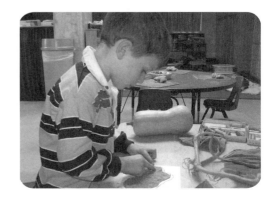

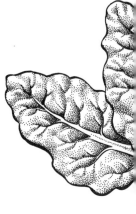

Lemony Swiss Chard Pasta

ESTIMATED TIME: 40 MINUTES

RECIPE
Yields about 18 servings
For this recipe, you will need these items:

FOOD INGREDIENTS
1 pound whole-wheat pasta
Medium-sized bunch of Swiss chard
Juice from 1 large or 2 small lemons
¼ teaspoon salt
¼ teaspoon pepper
2 tablespoons extra virgin olive oil
½ pound (8 ounces) feta cheese

SUPPLIES AND EQUIPMENT
Large pot
Measuring spoons
Cutting board
Plastic child-sized knives or kitchen scissors
Long wooden spoon
Wire whisk
Large mixing bowl

PROCEDURE

1. Bring a pot of water to a boil. When it's boiling, add the pasta to the pot and cook for 10 minutes until *al dente*, or just tender, stirring occasionally.

2. Meanwhile, wash the Swiss chard, remove its stems, and cut its leaves into small, ¹/3- to ½-inch pieces.

3. Squeeze the lemon juice into a large bowl, and remove any seeds from the juice.

4. To make the dressing, whisk together in the bowl lemon juice, salt, pepper, and olive oil.

5. Chop the feta into small pieces.

6. When the pasta is cooked add to the bowl pasta, chard, feta, and dressing.

7. Toss until well combined.

8. Serve family style and enjoy!

Suggested Ways to Involve Preschool Children in Cooking Activity:

☙ Children wash their hands and sit or stand around activity table. Announce, "Today we are going to make a recipe called Lemony Swiss Chard Pasta."

☙ Introduce and briefly describe each ingredient as you place it on the activity table: pasta, Swiss chard, lemons, salt, pepper, olive oil, and feta.

☙ Invite children to help wash the chard. Using child-sized knives or kitchen scissors, children can cut the chard and feta into small pieces.

☙ Cut the lemon into small wedges and invite children to help squeeze the lemon juice into the large bowl and whisk the dressing together.

☙ To combine ingredients, children can help measure and pour ingredients. One child can stir with the wooden spoon while others hold the bowl steady.

☙ Children will enjoy helping stir the pasta salad together until well combined.

☙ As always, remember to keep children away from all sharp cutting utensils, electrical devices, and hot food and surfaces at all times!

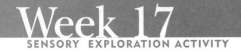

Carrots

ESTIMATED TIME: 30 MINUTES TO 1 HOUR

PURPOSE
To provide children with winter uses of carrots and ways to preserve carrots,

- Gather children and review the carrot with them. What do children remember from growing and harvesting the carrots? What part of the carrot do we eat?

- Explain the necessity of drying vegetables and how to use dried vegetables outside the growing cycle—for example, as carrot chips and dried carrot for soups.

- Provide children with blanched carrots, cutting boards, and child-sized kitchen knives. Remind them to use knives safely as they cut the carrots into chips.

- Ask children what will happen when they dry the carrots. What will happen to the juice? Do they remember what happened to the tomatoes when they were dried?

For this activity, you will need these items:

- Photo of carrots
- 5 or 6 child-sized plastic knives
- 1 bunch of carrots

- 5 or 6 cutting boards
- Large bowl to collect pieces
- Dehydrator

Note: This sensory activity requires cooking prior to the lesson. Cut carrots in half and then lengthwise. Place the carrot pieces in a pot of boiling water for 8 minutes. Cool the carrots prior to letting the children cut them.

PROCEDURE

1. Heat the oven to 140° F.

2. Children wash their hands and sit at the activity table. When all children are sitting, teacher hands out the knives. Children use knives safely to cut carrot chips.

3. Teacher(s) assists children as needed.

4. Teacher(s) asks children guiding questions.

5. After the carrot chips are placed on baking sheet, have an adult put the sheet in the preheated oven and dry the carrot chips for 4 to 8 hours. Or use a dehydrator set between 135° F and 140° F. Space the carrot chips 1 inch apart and dry them for 9 to 12 hours or until dried.

6. If children are interested, they can taste carrots and discuss texture and taste. Remind children to wash their hands again if they want to resume cutting carrots.

7. Clean up.

Carrot Sticks with Vanilla Dip

ESTIMATED TIME: 15 MINUTES

RECIPE

Yields about 18 servings
For this recipe, you will need these items:

FOOD INGREDIENTS

Small bag baby carrots (or 2 cups)
2 cups vanilla low-fat yogurt
1 teaspoon cinnamon

SUPPLIES AND EQUIPMENT

Mixing spoon
Large bowl
Measuring cups and spoons

PROCEDURE

1. Mix vanilla low-fat yogurt and cinnamon together.

2. Serve the yogurt mixture as a dip with the carrots.

Suggested Ways to Involve Preschool Children in Cooking Activity:

☙ Children wash their hands and sit or stand around the activity table. Announce, "Today we are going to make Carrot Sticks with Vanilla Dip."

☙ Each child can help measure and mix the ingredients in the dip.

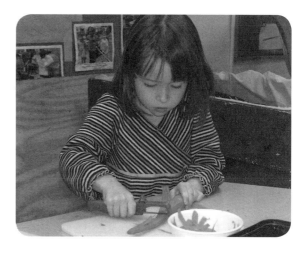

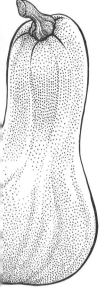

Butternut Squash

ESTIMATED TIME: 30 MINUTES TO 1 HOUR

PURPOSE

**To provide children with winter uses of butternut squash
and ways to preserve butternut squash,**

🌱 Gather children and review the butternut squash with them. Using a photo of butternut squash, ask the children what they remember from growing and harvesting butternut squash in the garden.

🌱 Provide children with child-sized graters, cutting boards, and raw butternut squash pieces that have been peeled and seeded. Remind children to use graters safely as they grate the squash pieces.

🌱 Ask children what the raw shredded squash tastes like and compare it to a cooked version they have tried before.

For this activity, you will need these items:

🌱 photo of butternut squash

🌱 5 or 6 child-sized graters

🌱 5 or 6 cutting boards

🌱 1 peeled and deseeded butternut squash cut in large chunks

🌱 Large bowl to collect grated pieces

🌱 Dehydrator

PROCEDURE

1. Children wash their hands and sit at the activity table. When all children are sitting, teacher hands out the graters. Children use graters safely to shred the squash pieces.

2. Teacher(s) assists children as needed.

3. Invite children to taste the shredded squash and discuss its taste and texture.

4. Remind children to wash their hands again if they want to resume grating squash. Extra grated squash can be used for the upcoming recipe.

5. Grated squash may be dried in the dehydrator by setting the dehydrator between 135° F and 140° F. Space the grated squash around and dry them for 9 to 12 hours or until dried.

6. Clean up.

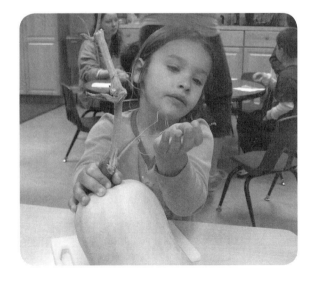

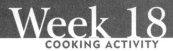

Butternut Squash Muffins

ESTIMATED TIME: 20 MINUTES, PLUS 20 TO 25 MINUTES BAKING TIME

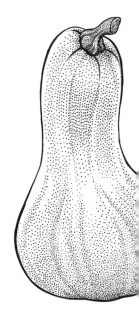

RECIPE
Yields 12 muffins
For this recipe, you will need these items:

FOOD INGREDIENTS
2 cups peeled, grated butternut squash
2 cups white whole-wheat flour
¾ cup low-fat milk
2 eggs
¼ cup canola oil
½ teaspoon salt
¼ cup brown sugar, packed
3 tablespoons pure maple syrup
2 teaspoons baking powder
1 teaspoon cinnamon
Nonstick cooking spray

SUPPLIES AND EQUIPMENT
Muffin pan (12 portions) and oven
Measuring cups and spoons
Grater
Large wooden spoon
Medium and large bowls
Toothpicks

PROCEDURE

1. Heat the oven to 350° F.

2. Spray the muffin tin with nonstick cooking spray.

3. In a medium bowl, stir together the grated squash, brown sugar, and maple syrup. Let the mixture sit for 10 minutes.

4. In a large bowl, combine flour, baking powder, cinnamon, and salt.

5. Add the squash mixture to the flour mixture. Add the remaining ingredients: milk, egg, and canola oil. Stir until the flour mixture is fully moistened. Do not overmix.

6. Spoon the batter into the prepared muffin cups, filling each well about two-thirds.

7. Bake the muffins for 20 to 25 minutes or until a toothpick inserted into the center of a muffin comes out clean.

Suggested Ways to Involve Preschool Children in Cooking Activity:

❦ Children wash their hands and gather around the activity table. Announce, "Today we are going to make a recipe called Butternut Squash Muffins."

❦ While the oven is preheating, have a couple of children spray the muffin pan lightly.

❦ Children can help measure and pour the ingredients into the bowls.

❦ When the ingredients have been measured, allow everyone a turn mixing the ingredients together, being careful not to overmix the batter lest it become tough.

❦ At a safe distance from the oven, allow children to observe while an adult places the muffin pan in the oven. If it can be done safely, allow children to watch the rising muffins.

❦ As always, remember to keep children away from all sharp cutting utensils, electrical devices, and hot food and surfaces at all times!

Other Indoor Winter Activities

Here are additional activities you can include in your classroom during these six weeks.

- ❦ Use children's literature to further explore garden and vegetable themes.

- ❦ *The Carrot Seed* by Ruth Krauss, with pictures by Crockett Johnson. Read the story and comment on the themes of the growing cycle and the giant carrot.

- ❦ *Stone Soup* retold by Heather Forest. Read the story and invite families to participate in a Stone Soup feast. Ask each child to bring one vegetable to the class. Then create a soup to serve to families at lunch.

- ❦ Provide props for vegetable gardening, a farmers' market, or a garden supply store in the dramatic play area. Include such items as seed packets, straw hats, a cash register, fruit and vegetable containers, plastic flowerpots, plastic or wooden vegetables, and child-sized plastic shovels.

- ❦ Use a planting and growing theme while you encourage children to become the six target vegetables at circle time. Begin by having children become seeds, curling their bodies on the floor. Add some nutrient-rich soil, water, and sun. Then have the seedlings sprout slowly toward the sun, stretching their bodies as they move upward. Ask each child which target vegetable he has grown to be. Remind the child to try to take the shape of that mature vegetable: a root in the ground (carrot), a leaf swaying in the breeze (chard), a large fruit or vegetable lying on the ground among leaves and vines (butternut squash), a fruit or vegetable hanging on vines and branches (cherry tomatoes, bell peppers), a fruit or vegetable reaching around the pole and hanging among the leaves (green beans).

ELEVEN

Spring Is Coming

Seeds and Planting Activities

WEEKS 19–24

THIS PART OF THE CURRICULUM ENCOURAGES a review of prior activities and concentrates experiences on seeds and the six target vegetables, as well as garden preparation. In some cases, we can dissect the vegetable and find the seeds. In other cases, we need to use packaged seeds (chard) or plant parts (carrots) to explore the beginning of the growing process. The seed activities promote:

- ❦ Understanding where seeds come from and how they are gathered
- ❦ Numeracy skills, such as counting and comparison of seeds
- ❦ Planting seeds and observing the beginning of the growing process

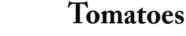

Tomatoes

ESTIMATED TIME: 30 MINUTES TO 1 HOUR

PURPOSE
To investigate seeds in preparation for the planting cycle,

- Gather children and review the tomato with them. Have them remind you about the plant's parts.

- How does a tomato grow? What part is planted?

- Provide children with cherry and large tomatoes, cutting boards, and child-sized knives. Prior to cutting the tomatoes, ask the children what is inside a tomato. Will the seeds be the same size in both of these tomatoes?

- Remind children to use the knives safely as they cut the tomatoes.

- Ask children to compare the seeds and to try to separate the seeds. Keep the seeds on a plate for drying and investigating later.

For this activity, you will need these items:

- 5 or 6 child-sized knives

- A quarter to a half large tomato and a half cherry tomato for each child

- 5 or 6 cutting boards

- Plate for seed storage

- Large bowl for tomato pieces

PROCEDURE

1. Children wash their hands and sit at the activity table. When all children are sitting, the teacher hands out the knives. Children use knives safely to cut tomatoes.

2. Teacher(s) assists children as needed.

3. Teacher(s) asks children to place tomato seeds on the plate for drying. Take time to look at the seeds, perhaps with a magnifying glass. Save these seeds for later exploration.

4. If children are interested, let them taste tomatoes and use descriptive words to compare the tastes of large and small tomatoes.

5. Remind children to wash their hands again if they want to resume cutting tomatoes.

6. Clean up.

Note: Save the dry seeds for the future activities listed at the end of this chapter. Dry seeds can be stored in a sealed plastic bag.

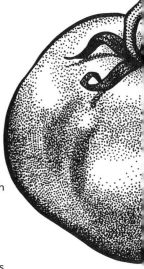

Tomato and Cheese Quesadillas

ESTIMATED TIME: 20 MINUTES, PLUS 15 MINUTES BAKING TIME

RECIPE

Yields 32 quesadilla slices
For this recipe, you will need these items:

FOOD INGREDIENTS

4 medium tomatoes, washed
2 cups shredded Monterey Jack cheese
8 medium whole-wheat tortillas or wraps
Nonstick cooking spray
Optional: salsa, low-fat sour cream,
    and/or guacamole

SUPPLIES AND EQUIPMENT

Cutting board, chef's knife for teacher
Plastic child-sized knives with small teeth
Small plates, one for each child
2 medium baking sheets, oven mitt
2 medium mixing bowls, serving plate
Oven for baking
Spatula for removing from baking sheets

PROCEDURE

1. Heat the oven to 400° F.

2. Wash the tomatoes and cut them into thick slices.

3. Lightly coat the baking sheets with nonstick cooking spray.

4. Place two tortillas on each sheet. Sprinkle shredded cheese evenly over the tortillas. Top each tortilla with a single layer of to-mato slices. Cover the quesadillas with the remaining tortillas.

5. Lightly mist the tops of the quesadillas with nonstick cooking spray. Bake them in the heated oven for approximately 15 minutes.

6. Allow the quesadilla to cool, then cut them into fourths. Transfer the slices to a serving plate. Serve them family style with salsa, low-fat sour cream, and/or guacamole, if desired. Enjoy!

Suggested Ways to Involve Preschool Children in Cooking Activity:

❦ Children wash their hands and sit or stand around the activity table. Announce, "Today we are going to make Tomato and Cheese Quesadillas."

❦ Introduce all ingredients needed for the recipe: tomatoes, tortillas, and cheese.

❦ Ask children to rinse the tomatoes in the sink. Have them practice cutting the toma-toes, using the child-sized knives while work-ing over the small plates.

❦ Invite children to sprinkle the shredded cheese onto the tortillas. Demonstrate and then encourage them to top the cheese with a layer of tomato slices.

❦ Show an older child how to hold the cook-ing spray 6 to 8 inches away and use a gentle sweeping motion to coat the baking sheets. Younger children may then place the tortillas on the sheets.

❦ As always, remember to keep children away from all sharp cutting utensils, electrical devices, and hot food and surfaces at all times!

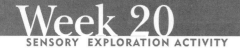

Green Beans

ESTIMATED TIME: 30 MINUTES TO 1 HOUR

PURPOSE

To investigate seeds in preparation for the planting cycle,

- Gather children and review the green bean with them. Ask them to remind you about the plant's parts.

- How does a green bean grow? What part is planted?

- Provide children with green beans, cutting boards, and child-sized knives. Prior to cutting the green beans, ask children what is inside the bean pod. Remind children to use knives safely as they cut the green beans lengthwise.

- Ask children to scoop out and separate the seeds. Keep seeds on a plate for drying and investigating later.

- Show children the kidney bean and explain that it is a cousin of the green beans. Plant the bean in a moist paper towel and place bean and paper towel into a plastic bag (see procedure, step 6).

For this activity, you will need these items:

- 5 or 6 child-sized knives

- 2 or 3 green beans per child

- 5 or 6 cutting boards

- Plate for seed storage

- Large bowl for green bean pieces

- 1 kidney bean, wet paper towel, and a plastic bag (or one of each item for each child)

PROCEDURE

1. Children wash their hands and sit at the activity table. When all children are sitting, the teacher hands out the knives. Children use knives safely to cut green beans lengthwise.

2. Teacher(s) assists children as needed.

3. Teacher(s) asks children to place green bean seeds on a plate for drying. Take time to look at the seeds, perhaps with a magnifying glass. Save these seeds for a later exploration.

4. If children are interested, let them taste the green beans.

5. Remind children to wash their hands again if they want to resume cutting green beans.

6. Plant a kidney bean in the plastic bag and observe and record its growing cycle over several days. First soak kidney beans for several hours or even overnight. Take one sheet of a paper towel and wet it thoroughly. Place the bean and the wet paper towel in the plastic bag. Make sure the seed is visible and touching the paper towel. Place the bag near a window or tape it to the window where you and the children can easily complete your observations.

7. Clean up.

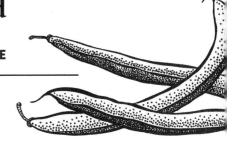

Green and Orange Pasta Salad

**ESTIMATED TIME: 20 TO 25 MINUTES,
PLUS AN OPTIONAL 30 MINUTES OF REFRIGERATOR TIME**

RECIPE
Yields about 18 servings
For this recipe, you will need these items:

FOOD INGREDIENTS
2 tablespoons balsamic vinegar
3 tablespoons olive oil
1 pound whole-grain pasta
1 pound green beans
6 carrots
1 cup shredded Parmesan cheese
Salt and pepper to taste

SUPPLIES AND EQUIPMENT
Large serving bowl, long wooden spoon
Measuring spoons and cups
Food processor for shredding carrots
Plastic or flatware child-sized knives
Chef's knife, cutting board for teacher
Vegetable steamer or skillet, strainer
Large pot, vegetable peeler

PROCEDURE

1. Bring a pot of water to boil for the pasta.

2. Wash the green beans and snap off their stems.

3. Cut or break the green beans into bite-sized pieces and place them in a steamer or a skillet filled with ¾ inch of water.

4. Steam or cook the green beans over high heat for 5 to 9 minutes or until tender. Cool the beans by rinsing them under cold water.

5. Wash and peel the carrots.

6. Shred the carrots in a food processor or dice them using a chef's knife.

7. When the water is boiling, put in the pasta and cook for 10 minutes, or until *al dente* (just tender). When pasta is done, drain it in the strainer. Rinse the strainer of pasta under cold water to cool it.

8. Combine in a large bowl: vinegar, oil, cheese, salt, and pepper. Then add: pasta, carrots, and green beans.

9. Mix until all the ingredients are evenly combined.

10. Serve immediately, or store in refrigerator for 30 minutes to cool further.

Suggested Ways to Involve Preschool Children in Cooking Activity:

❦ Children wash their hands and sit or stand around the activity table. Announce, "Today we are going to use green beans and carrots to make a recipe called Green and Orange Pasta Salad."

❦ Introduce and briefly describe each ingredient for the recipe as you place it on the activity table.

❦ To prepare the green beans, invite children to wash the beans, snap off their stems, and cut or snap the beans into small pieces.

❦ To prepare the carrots, children can help wash the carrots.

❦ Children enjoy watching you process the carrots.

❦ To combine ingredients, older children (four- to five-year-olds) can measure and younger children (two- to three-year-olds) can pour the ingredients.

❦ Children enjoy mixing the pasta salad ingredients together.

❦ As always, remember to keep children away from all sharp cutting utensils, electrical devices, and hot food and surfaces at all times!

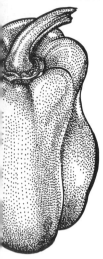

Bell Peppers

ESTIMATED TIME: 30 MINUTES TO 1 HOUR

PURPOSE
To investigate seeds in preparation for the planting cycle,

🌱 Gather children and review the bell pepper with them. Ask them to remind you about the plant parts.

🌱 How does a green pepper grow? What part is planted? How are different colored bell peppers grown?

🌱 Provide children with a quarter bell pepper, cutting boards, and child-sized knives. Prior to cutting the bell peppers, ask children what is inside the pepper. Remind children

to use knives safely as they cut the bell peppers and remove the seeds.

🌱 Ask children to scoop and separate the seeds. Keep the seeds on a plate for drying and investigating later.

🌱 Show children the tomato, bean, and pepper seeds together. What words can they use to describe the seeds? Can they match the seeds to the photos of the vegetables?

For this activity, you will need these items:

🌱 5 or 6 child-sized knives

🌱 Half a bell pepper per child

🌱 5 or 6 cutting boards

🌱 Plate for seed storage

🌱 Large bowl for the bell pepper pieces

🌱 Seeds, such as tomato or green bean seeds, from previous activities

🌱 Tomato, bean, and bell pepper photos or pictures from magazines or seed catalogs

PROCEDURE

1. Children wash their hands and sit at the activity table. When all children are sitting, the teacher hands out the knives. Children use knives safely to cut bell peppers and remove seeds.

2. Teacher(s) assists children as needed.

3. Teacher(s) asks children to place the bell pepper seeds on a plate for drying. Take time to look at the seeds, perhaps with a

magnifying glass. Save these seeds for a later exploration.

4. If children are interested, let them taste the bell peppers.

5. Remind children to wash their hands again if they want to resume cutting bell peppers.

6. Provide children with seeds from previous activities to look at and compare.

7. Clean up.

Note: Save the dry seeds for the future activities listed at the end of this chapter. Dry seeds can be stored in a sealed plastic bag.

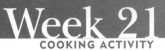

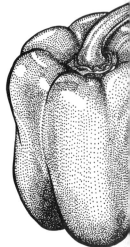

Bell Pepper and Pineapple Fried Rice

ESTIMATED TIME: 30 MINUTES

RECIPE

Yields about 18 servings
For this recipe, you will need these items:

FOOD INGREDIENTS

2 bell peppers
½ cup crushed pineapple in own juice
4 cups cooked brown or basmati rice
3 tablespoons vegetable oil
2 cloves fresh garlic (1 teaspoon crushed)
1 small piece fresh ginger root
   (2 teaspoons grated), plus section
   for children to examine
2 tablespoons low-sodium tamari
   (wheat-free soy sauce)

SUPPLIES AND EQUIPMENT

Food processor, manual can opener
Cheese grater, handheld garlic press
Large wok or skillet with heat source
Measuring cups and spoons
Cutting board, chef's knife for teachers
Large wooden spoon or spatula
Small plates, one for each child
Plastic or flatware child-sized knives
Serving platter and large spoon
Rice cooker or pot, strainer

PROCEDURE

1. Precook the 1⅓ cups of rice in 2⅔ cups water. (This will take 35 to 45 minutes.)

2. Wash the bell peppers and remove their seeds. Finely chop the bell peppers.

3. Peel the ginger and finely grate it using the cheese grater or finely dice it with a knife.

4. Remove the outer skin from the garlic and crush the cloves in a garlic press or finely mince the garlic cloves using a knife.

5. In the following order, add to preheated wok or skillet at medium heat: oil, peppers, 1 teaspoon ginger, and 1 teaspoon garlic.

6. Raise the burner heat to medium-high and sauté peppers, ginger, and garlic until the peppers are soft. Add the rice and pineapple.

7. Gently stir the rice mixture using a wooden spoon or spatula, moving ingredients around to disperse the oil and flavorings. Add the tamari and continue to heat for an additional 1 to 2 minutes.

8. When the rice mixture is evenly heated and combined, remove the pan from heat, uncover, and stir lightly.

9. Allow the rice to cool slightly. Transfer it to a serving platter. Serve family style and enjoy!

Suggested Ways to Involve Preschool Children in Cooking Activity:

🌱 Children wash their hands and sit or stand around the activity table. Announce, "Today we are going to make Bell Pepper and Pineapple Fried Rice."

🌱 Children can help with washing the vegetables, removing their seeds, and rough chopping them. You can later chop them more finely using a sharp knife.

🌱 Show children what the ginger root looks like whole. Explain that ginger root grows underground like a carrot does. Grate one end and pass the root around so children can smell the ginger.

🌱 Because the ingredients are added to the skillet or wok while it is still cool, children can perform this step themselves. Let them take turns measuring and pouring each ingredient listed. Just make sure that the oil goes in first so it will get hot enough to fry the rice and vegetables when you turn on the burner.

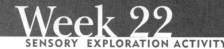

Swiss Chard

ESTIMATED TIME: 30 MINUTES TO 1 HOUR

PURPOSE
To investigate seeds in preparation for the planting cycle,

- ❦ Gather children and review Swiss chard with them. Ask them to remind you about the plant's parts.

- ❦ How does the chard grow? What part is planted? What are some colors of rainbow chard?

- ❦ Provide children with packaged Swiss chard seeds, Swiss chard leaves, cutting boards, and child-sized kitchen scissors.

- ❦ Ask children to investigate the chard seeds. Keep the seeds on a plate for planting. Perhaps use a magnifying glass to observe the seeds. What shape are the seeds? How big or small are they compared to other target vegetable seeds you've observed?

MATERIALS

- ❦ 5 or 6 child-sized kitchen scissors
- ❦ Half a chard leaf per child
- ❦ 5 or 6 cutting boards
- ❦ Small planting pot for each child

- ❦ Potting soil
- ❦ Swiss chard seeds
- ❦ Large bowl for leaf pieces

PROCEDURE

1. Children wash their hands and sit at the activity table. When all children are sitting, the teacher hands out the kitchen scissors. Children use scissors to safely cut the chard. If desired, save cut chard for the cooking activity later in the week.

2. Teacher(s) assists children as needed.

3. Teacher(s) asks children to place the chard in a bowl.

4. If children are interested, let them taste the chard pieces.

5. Remind children to wash their hands again if they want to resume cutting chard. Provide children with planting cups, soil, and chard seeds. Plant the seeds by filling each cup three-quarters full with potting soil. Place a seed on the soil and cover it with about a quarter inch of soil. Add water until the soil is moist. Keep the cups at room temperature. Keep the soil moist until a sprout appears above the surface. After the seeds sprout, place the cups in a spot that receives direct sunlight for at least 6 hours per day. Continue to water as necessary to keep soil moist. Watch them grow.

6. Clean up.

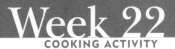

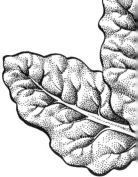

Cheesy Swiss Chard Squares

ESTIMATED TIME: 30 MINUTES, PLUS 25 TO 30 MINUTES FOR BAKING

RECIPE
Yields about 18 squares
For this recipe, you will need these items:

FOOD INGREDIENTS
4 slices whole-wheat bread
½ pound fresh Swiss chard
4 eggs
2 teaspoons vegetable oil
½ cup grated Parmesan cheese
½ cup shredded mozzarella cheese
Salt and pepper to taste
Nonstick cooking spray

SUPPLIES AND EQUIPMENT
Toaster, whisk
Cutting board, chef's knife for teacher
Plastic child-sized knives or kitchen scissors
Skillet with heat source
Large mixing bowl
Casserole dish
Mixing spoons, measuring cups
Oven, oven mitt
Spatula
Serving dish and plates

PROCEDURE

1. Heat the oven to 350° F.

2. Toast the bread in a toaster. Allow the slices to cool and then cut or tear them into very small cubes.

3. Wash the chard, remove its stems, and chop or tear the leaves into small pieces.

4. Cook the chard in 2 teaspoons of vegetable oil in a covered skillet over medium heat for 4 to 5 minutes. Drain excess liquid.

5. Whisk the eggs in a large mixing bowl.

6. Add to the eggs and stir until well combined: chard, bread, cheese, salt, and pepper.

7. Lightly coat a casserole dish with the cooking spray.

8. Place mixture in the casserole dish.

9. Bake for 25 to 30 minutes. Allow to cool and then cut into small square servings.

10. Serve and enjoy.

Suggested Ways to Involve Preschool Children in Cooking Activity:

☙ Children wash their hands and sit or stand around the activity table. Announce, "Today we are going to make a recipe called Cheesy Swiss Chard Squares."

☙ Introduce and briefly describe the origin of each ingredient for the recipe as you place it on the activity table.

☙ After toasting the bread slices, invite children to help cut or tear the bread into very small pieces.

☙ To prepare the chard, invite children to help wash the leaves, remove the stems, and cut the chard leaves into small pieces.

☙ To combine ingredients, older children (four- to five-year-olds) can measure and younger children (two- to three-year-olds) can pour wet and dry ingredients into the mixing bowl.

☙ Children can take turns stirring the mixture.

☙ Children can help transfer the ingredients from the mixing bowl to the casserole dish.

☙ As always, remember to keep children away from all sharp cutting utensils, electrical devices, and hot food and surfaces at all times!

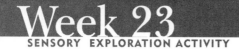

Carrots

ESTIMATED TIME: 30 MINUTES TO 1 HOUR

PURPOSE
**To provide a relationship between the harvesting of carrots
from the garden and growing the carrot tops,**

❦ How did we harvest the carrots from our garden beds? Did we pick them from a plant? What part of the carrot do we eat? Where does the orange part of the carrot grow? Where are the seeds of the carrot?

❦ If available, bring in Queen Anne's lace to observe and investigate wild carrot seeds.

For this activity, you will need these items:

❦ 5 or 6 child-sized knives

❦ 5 or 6 cutting boards

❦ 1 growing dish, or an aluminum pie plate with water-soaked paper towels

❦ 1 storage tray

❦ 1 bunch of carrots with tops

❦ 1 grater

PROCEDURE

1. Children wash their hands and sit at the activity table. When all children are sitting, the teacher hands out the knives. Children cut tops off carrots if they are able; otherwise, teacher cuts off tops, including about one-half inch of the root, including the carrot greens.

2. Children arrange the carrot tops on the pie plate on top of the soaked paper towel and set the plate aside to observe the carrot greens' growth. Water needs to be visible in the pan and the paper towel soaking wet for the tops to continue to grow or stay fresh.

3. Provide children with half a carrot each to grate in preparation for this week's Carrot Muffins recipe. Offer children tastes if they want them. Remind children to wash their hands after eating if they want to resume grating.

4. Clean up.

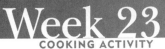

Carrot Muffins

ESTIMATED TIME: 35 TO 40 MINUTES

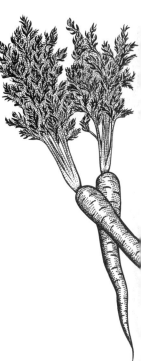

RECIPE
Yields 12 muffins
For this recipe, you will need these items:

FOOD INGREDIENTS

1½ cups white whole-wheat flour
1 teaspoon baking powder
1 teaspoon baking soda, ¼ teaspoon salt
2 teaspoons ground cinnamon
¾ cup maple syrup, ¼ cup orange juice
1½ cups packed finely shredded carrots
5 tablespoons canola oil, 2 large eggs
½ cup golden raisins
Nonstick cooking spray

SUPPLIES AND EQUIPMENT

Standard 12-muffin pan
Measuring spoons and cups
Long wooden spoon
Food processor for shredding carrots
Wire whisk
Medium mixing bowl
Large mixing bowl
Toothpicks
Oven mitts

PROCEDURE

1. Heat the oven to 400° F.

2. Lightly spray a standard 12-muffin pan with nonstick cooking spray.

3. Wash the carrots and shred them in the food processor.

4. In a medium bowl, whisk together the eggs and maple syrup.

5. Stir in shredded carrots, orange juice, golden raisins, and vegetable oil.

6. In a large bowl, combine flour, baking powder, baking soda, cinnamon, and salt.

7. Create a well, or indentation, in the middle of the dry ingredients. Slowly add the liquid ingredients to it. Mix just until the dry ingredients are moistened. It is important not to overmix.

8. Spoon the muffin batter into muffin molds until each is two-thirds full. Bake the muffins for about 20 minutes or until a toothpick inserted into the centers comes out clean.

9. Allow the muffins to cool before you serve them.

Suggested Ways to Involve Preschool Children in Cooking Activity:

- Children wash their hands and sit or stand around the activity table. Announce, "Today we are going to make a recipe called Carrot Muffins using carrots like the ones we grew last summer."

- Introduce and briefly describe each ingredient as you place it on the activity table. For example, explain that golden raisins are actually dried green grapes.

- Children may enjoy watching you shred the carrots. They can push the food processor's *on* button.

- To combine ingredients, older children (four- to five-year-olds) can measure and younger children (two- to three-year-olds) can pour the ingredients. One child can stir the mixture with the wooden spoon while others hold the bowl steady.

- Children enjoy cracking the eggs and later spooning the final mixture into the muffin cups.

- As always, remember to keep children away from all sharp cutting utensils, electrical devices, and hot food and surfaces at all times!

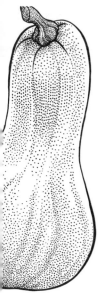

Butternut Squash

ESTIMATED TIME: 30 MINUTES TO 1 HOUR

PURPOSE

To investigate seeds in preparation for the planting cycle,

❦ Gather children and review the squash plant with them. Ask them to remind you about the plant's parts.

❦ How does a butternut squash grow? What part is planted?

❦ Provide children with cooked squash, cutting boards, and child-sized knives. Before cutting the squash, ask children what is inside the squash.

❦ Remind children to use knives safely as they cut the squash.

❦ Ask children to scoop and separate the seeds. Keep the seeds on a plate for drying and investigating later.

For this activity, you will need these items:

❦ 5 or 6 child-sized knives

❦ 1 or 2 cooked squashes for each group of 6 children

❦ 5 or 6 cutting boards

❦ Plate for seed storage

❦ Large bowl for squash pieces

❦ Waxed paper

Note: This sensory activity requires cooking prior to the lesson. Cut the squash in half lengthwise, scoop out the seeds, place the squash halves in a shallow pan of water, and bake them for 50 minutes or until very tender.

PROCEDURE

1. Children wash their hands and sit at the activity table. When all children are sitting, teacher hands out the knives. Children use knives safely to cut squash.

2. Teacher(s) assists the children as needed.

3. Teacher(s) asks children to place squash seeds on plate for drying. Take time to look at the seeds, perhaps with a magnifying glass.

4. Invite children to taste the squash.

5. Remind children to wash their hands again if they want to resume cutting squash

6. Rinse the seeds and place them on waxed paper for drying.

7. Compare the dried seeds with other seeds collected from previous activities.

8. Clean up.

Note: Save the dried seeds for the future activities listed at the end of this chapter. Dried seeds can be stored in a sealed plastic bag.

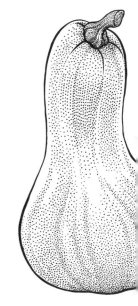

Butternut Squash Fries

ESTIMATED TIME: 30 MINUTES, PLUS 20 MINUTES BAKING TIME

RECIPE

Yields about 18 servings
For this recipe, you will need these items:

FOOD INGREDIENTS

2 medium butternut squash, lightly
steamed, peeled, and cut into large
chunks, seeds left intact
Salt
Nonstick cooking spray

SUPPLIES AND EQUIPMENT

2 baking sheets, spoons
Small plates, one per child
Plastic or flatware child-sized knives
Chef's knife and cutting board
Spatula for cooking

PROCEDURE

1. Heat the oven to 425° F.

2. Peel and cut up squash into large chunks, leaving seeds intact. Place the squash chunks in the steamer and lightly steam, checking for tenderness occasionally. Do not overcook the squash. Cool squash.

3. Use spoons to scoop and remove the seeds.

4. Cut the steamed squash chunks into long, thin, french-fry shapes.

5. Place the squash fries on baking sheets that have been sprayed with nonstick cooking spray. Sprinkle the fries lightly with salt.

6. Place the baking sheets in the preheated oven and bake for 20 minutes or so, turning fries over halfway through baking process. Fries are done when they start to brown on the edges and become crispy.

7. Serve alone or with a favorite condiment or dip.

Suggested Ways to Involve Preschool Children in Cooking Activity:

🍴 Have children wash their hands and then announce, "Today we are going to make Butternut Squash Fries using butternut squash."

🍴 Enlist children in spraying the baking sheets with nonstick cooking spray.

🍴 Show children how they can help remove the remaining seeds by using their plastic knives to gently scrape them onto a plate or into a compost container.

🍴 Allow each child to have a medium piece of squash on a small plate. Guide children in cutting the squash into french-fry-shaped pieces, using the child-sized knives. Cut any remaining pieces of squash into fries.

🍴 After the squash have been cut into fries, let children gently lay their fries onto one of the baking sheets. Have children count their fries as they do this: "One squash fry, two squash fries, three squash fries. . . ."

🍴 Before placing the fries in the oven, mention how the squash fries look and describe how they will change color after baking to look brown and crispy.

🍴 At a safe distance from the oven, allow children to look at the fries when they are done so they can distinguish the browned and crispy-looking fries from slightly cooked fries. Remind children how the fries looked before baking.

🍴 As always, remember to keep children away from all sharp cutting utensils, electrical devices, and hot food and surfaces at all times!

Other Seed and Planting Activities

Here are additional activities you can include in your classroom during these six weeks:

- Use dried seeds to create musical shakers. Decorate a paper tube, tape construction paper over its bottom using masking tape, and make sure the fit is secure. Add seeds to the tube and tape the top closed using construction paper and masking tape. Or place a collection of the dried seeds in a small plastic container with a cover. Children can decorate the container with stickers.

- Glue dried seeds on paper that has been cut out in the shape of a vegetable, so the pepper seeds are glued to the paper that is the pepper shape and color, the butternut squash seeds are glued to paper in a butternut squash shape and color, and so on.

- Glue an assortment of the seeds on brown paper for a collage.

- Try to plant the dried seeds in small potting planters or peat planters and observe what happens.

~ TWELVE ~

THE FAMILY RECIPE KITS

As part of the Early Sprouts curriculum, we prepare Family Recipe Kits to send home each week. Each kit contains a recipe, a feedback questionnaire, and some of the ingredients, measured and packed for ease of use.

The purpose of the Family Recipe Kit is to provide a healthy recipe that family members can easily prepare at home with their child. The program helps busy families at the end of the week by providing many of the ingredients used in the kit recipe. Each week of the curriculum offers a version of the featured recipe for families to prepare at home, reduced in size to the portions appropriate for a family—also keeping the costs of the kits reasonable. Ideally, Family Recipe Kits are sent home at the end of each week throughout the twenty-four-week program. This way families have many opportunities to explore the target vegetables themselves. Additional exposures to the vegetables have a positive impact on the child and other family members. (For more on the impact of this component of the program on families, see chapter 13.)

We recognize that early childhood centers have budgetary and time constraints; therefore, we encourage you to send home as many Family Recipe Kits as feasible during the program. The family-sized recipes do help minimize costs, preparation time, and materials needed to assemble the kits. Another option is to look for additional funding to support this aspect of the program. We have received grant funding from various sources to help finance the food items included in the Family Recipe Kits and have found volunteers to help prepare the kits. If sending home the recipe kits is not possible, we recommend that you provide families with a copy of the weekly recipe as a way to share the program with them.

Supplies Needed

This equipment and these materials are needed to prepare the Family Recipe Kits to go home:

- ❦ 2-ounce, 4-ounce, and 8-ounce plastic containers with tight-fitting lids (available at restaurant supply stores)
- ❦ Plastic bags in snack, sandwich, and quart sizes
- ❦ Larger bags for children to transport all of the ingredients*
- ❦ Recipes and ingredients
- ❦ Family feedback questionnaire, customized for your program and for each recipe (see the questionnaire template, page 140)
- ❦ A few baskets or small boxes to hold individual ingredients for in-class packing.

Grocery stores may be willing to donate cloth bags to early childhood programs for use with the Early Sprouts program.

Packing the Family Recipe Kits

On the day when a Family Recipe Kit is going to be sent home, a staff member or volunteer needs time to prepare the ingredients for the week's recipe. The actual time depends on the number of children and families and the number of ingredients

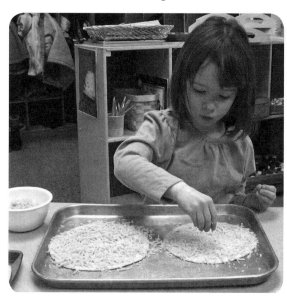

the specific recipe requires. Each ingredient should be measured and packaged separately. The exception to this is the dry ingredients for a muffin, cookie, or cake recipe, which we do combine. We do not send home such items as vegetable oil, salt, pepper, milk, or eggs. The liquids listed here are likely to spill or leak on the way home, and fragile ingredients, such as eggs, may break. Our participating families have assured us that these items are available in their home kitchen or pantry. Each family recipe specifies the ingredients included in the prep kit and those needed from the home kitchen.

After the ingredients have been measured and packaged, place each ingredient in a separate container. We like to use baskets or small boxes to hold the packaged ingredients. Copies of the featured recipe and the feedback questionnaire should be neatly piled next to the ingredients. Cloth bags marked with children's names work well to carry the kit home. We recommend that you keep a supply of plastic or paper shopping bags on hand in case a family does not return the cloth bag promptly.

To include and help them take ownership of the process, children complete the final packing of the recipe kits. As they visit the packing table, they each gather one container or bag from each of the ingredients baskets. When children recognize the routine of this packing process, it becomes an exciting end-of-the-day activity. Packing the Family Recipe Kit helps promote children's cognitive development because they are working on reading and mathematical skills through this process!

It is best to send the Family Recipe Kits home toward the end of the week. That way the children are familiar with the vegetable that has been featured during the week. They have participated in sensory exploration and have had the opportunity to prepare the recipe. We prefer sending Family Recipe Kits home on Thursday so we have Friday as a backup to ensure that the kit goes home. It is important to pack the kits at the end of the day, because the recipe may include perishable ingredients that need to be kept cool. When children are absent, pack, label, and refrigerate their Family Recipe Kits. Be sure to remind parents that you are sending home an Early Sprouts Family Recipe Kit so the kit is not accidentally left in the car or backpack overnight. Colorful signs on the exit door and reminders by the sign-in list are effective for offering such reminders. Children often place a note in their cubbies to help families remember to take the kits home.

Each week, along with the recipe and materials sent home in the Family Recipe Kit, we include a brief questionnaire designed to gather feedback from families. A sample is provided on the following page.

Home-School Connection

Good communication and understanding between home and school enhance children's learning. Early childhood educators are always looking for positive ways to share what children are doing during the school day with their families. The Early Sprouts Family Recipe Kits are an excellent way to bring the Early Sprouts program and activities into the home. Our research results indicate an added benefit: the kits help change eating habits.

Early Sprouts Family Recipe Kit Questionnaire

Please circle your answer and return questionnaire to your child's classroom.

Did you prepare *(insert name of recipe)*, this week's take-home recipe?
Yes   No

If yes, did your preschool child help prepare the recipe?
Yes   No

Did your preschool child eat any of the prepared recipe?
Yes   No   Did not prepare

How much did your family like/dislike the recipe?
Liked
Neither disliked nor liked
Disliked
Do not know/did not prepare or try

Would you prepare the recipe again?
Yes   No   Maybe

Additional comments/feedback (optional):

Thank you for taking the time to complete the questionnaire.
Child's name (optional): _____

If you have any questions or comments about the Early Sprouts project that you would like to share, please contact *(insert your contact name, e-mail, and phone number)*.

We use the information gathered on these forms to informally assess families' impressions of the program. We also collect data on their participation and their children's involvement in preparing the kits at home. Family feedback has helped us adjust the recipes and to improve the program. In chapter 13, you will find more details about what we have learned from the family feedback.

Early Sprouts Family Recipe Kits

The following pages contain copies of the recipes that are sent home to families.

Recipe #	Name	Target Vegetable
1	Cherry Tomatoes with Honey Mustard Dip	Tomato
2	Chinese-Style Green Beans	Green Beans
3	Bell Pepper Couscous Castles	Bell Pepper
4	Cheddar and Chard Quesadillas	Swiss Chard
5	Carrot Oatmeal Cookies	Carrot
6	Butternut Squash Pancakes	Butternut Squash
7	Pasta with Garlic-Parmesan Tomato Sauce	Tomato
8	Green Bean Wontons with Dipping Sauce	Green Beans
9	Confetti Corn Muffins	Bell Pepper
10	Pita Pocket Pizzas	Swiss Chard
11	Honey Glazed Carrots	Carrot
12	Banana Squash Smoothie	Butternut Squash
13	English Muffin Pizzas with Homemade Sauce	Tomato
14	Sesame Seed Green Beans	Green Beans
15	Bell Pepper Veggie Burgers	Bell Pepper
16	Lemony Swiss Chard Pasta	Swiss Chard
17	Carrot Sticks with Vanilla Dip	Carrot
18	Butternut Squash Muffins	Butternut Squash
19	Tomato and Cheese Quesadillas	Tomato
20	Green and Orange Pasta Salad	Green Beans
21	Bell Pepper and Pineapple Fried Rice	Bell Pepper
22	Cheesy Swiss Chard Squares	Swiss Chard
23	Carrot Muffins	Carrot
24	Butternut Squash Fries	Butternut Squash

Note: If a family requests a recipe with a bigger yield, you can share the classroom version, which makes 6 entrée or 18 snack-sized servings.

Cherry Tomatoes with Honey Mustard Dip

ESTIMATED TIME: 15 MINUTES
Yields 4 servings

For this recipe, you will need these items:

INCLUDED IN THE RECIPE KIT:
½ pint of cherry tomatoes (10 to 12 tomatoes)
¼ cup low-fat or nonfat plain yogurt
1 teaspoon spicy brown mustard
1 teaspoon honey

Prepare the recipe by following these steps:

1. Wash cherry tomatoes, slice them in half, and set them aside.

2. Measure and place the yogurt, mustard, and honey in a medium bowl.

3. Stir until well mixed and smooth.

4. Pour the dressing into small dipping cups or bowls.

5. Enjoy cherry tomatoes dipped in honey mustard dressing.

Here are some ways to involve your children in cooking:

❧ Children can cut cherry tomatoes using a child-sized knife. Finish any incomplete cutting yourself.

❧ Older children can measure and younger children can pour the ingredients.

❧ Children can take turns stirring the dip until it is well mixed.

❧ Remember to keep children away from all sharp cutting equipment!

Note: If you prefer a recipe that yields 6 entrée servings or 18 snack-sized portions, please ask for the classroom version.

Nutrition Information Per Serving

22 calories	< 1 g total fat
0 g saturated fat	4 g carbohydrates
0.5 g fiber	3 g sugar
1 mg cholesterol	22 mg sodium

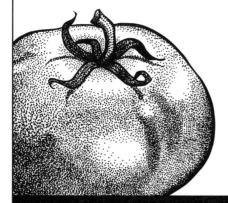

FAMILY RECIPE KIT

EARLY SPROUTS

Chinese-Style Green Beans

ESTIMATED TIME: 25 MINUTES
Yields 4 servings

For this recipe, you will need these items:

INCLUDED IN THE RECIPE KIT:
½ pound green beans
2 teaspoons unsalted butter
2 teaspoons low-sodium tamari
1 teaspoon fresh lemon juice (⅛ of
    lemon squeezed)

FROM YOUR KITCHEN:
2½ cups of water

Prepare the recipe by following these steps:

1. In a nonstick skillet, melt the butter over low heat on the stovetop. Place a medium pot of water on another burner and bring it to a boil.

2. Clean the green beans, remove their stems, and snap them in half.

3. When the butter has melted, remove it from the heat and use a wooden spoon to stir in the tamari and lemon juice. Set aside.

4. Add the green beans to the boiling water and boil for 5 minutes, or until tender.

5. Turn off the heat and drain green beans in a colander.

6. Add the green beans to the butter/tamari mixture and gently toss to combine.

Here are some ways to involve your children in cooking:

- Children can wash the beans, snap off their stems, and snap them in half.

- Older children can measure ingredients, and younger children can pour ingredients. Children can stir ingredients together.

- Remember to keep children away from sharp cutting utensils, electrical devices, and hot food and surfaces at all times!

Note: If you prefer a recipe that yields 6 entrée servings or 18 snack-sized portions, please ask for the classroom version.

Nutrition Information Per Serving

35 calories	2 g total fat
1 g saturated fat	4 g carbohydrates
2 g fiber	1 g sugar
5 mg cholesterol	154 mg sodium

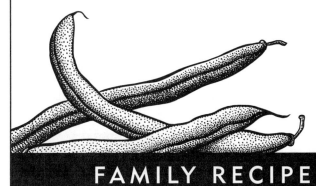

Bell Pepper Couscous Castles

ESTIMATED TIME: 25 MINUTES
Yields 8 small servings

For this recipe, you will need these items:

INCLUDED IN THE RECIPE KIT:
1 cup whole-wheat couscous
½ diced bell pepper
¼ cup (thawed) frozen corn
1 cup of vegetable broth

FROM YOUR KITCHEN:
Vegetable oil
Small pinch paprika (optional)
Ice cubes

Prepare the recipe by following these steps:

1. Clean the bell pepper, remove its seeds, and dice it into small pieces.

2. Coat a skillet with a small amount of vegetable oil. Add the diced bell pepper and the corn to the skillet. Raise the heat to medium-high and sauté the vegetables until they're tender.

3. Add the vegetable broth and couscous to the skillet. Cook, while stirring, about 5 minutes or until the broth has been absorbed. Remove skillet from the heat, cover, and let sit another minute or two.

4. Transfer the couscous and vegetables to a large mixing bowl and stir. Add ice cubes, one at a time, while stirring, until the mixture cools enough to handle.

5. Use the small plastic container the corn was packed in to pack the couscous mixture and then turn it upside down onto a small plate to create the castles. Makes about 8 castles.

6. If desired, lightly sprinkle the castles with paprika.

Here are some ways to involve your children in cooking:

- Children can help with washing, removing seeds, and rough-chopping the peppers, which you can then more finely chop with a sharp knife.

- The recipe allows the vegetables to be added to the skillet while it is still cold, so children can place the diced peppers into the oiled skillet and measure and pour in the corn.

- Children can stir the vegetables and couscous.

- When the couscous mixture is cool, you can place the mixing bowl on a table, and children can take the lead in making the sand castles.

- Remember to keep children away from sharp cutting utensils, electrical devices, and hot food and surfaces at all times!

Note: If you prefer a recipe that yields 6 entrée servings or 18 snack-sized portions, please ask for the classroom version.

Nutrition Information Per Serving

66 calories	1 g total fat
0 g saturated fat	13 g carbohydrates
2 g fiber	1 g sugar
0 mg cholesterol	118 mg sodium

Cheddar and Chard Quesadillas

ESTIMATED TIME: 20 MINUTES, PLUS 15 MINUTES BAKING TIME
Yields 4 servings

For this recipe, you will need these items:

INCLUDED IN THE RECIPE KIT:
1/3 pound of Swiss chard
1/2 cup shredded cheddar cheese
2 whole-wheat tortillas or wraps

FROM YOUR KITCHEN:
Nonstick cooking spray
Optional: low-fat sour cream, salsa, and/or guacamole

Prepare the recipe by following these steps:

1. Heat the oven to 400° F.

2. Wash the Swiss chard and remove its stems.

3. Cut or tear the chard into 2-inch pieces.

4. Heat a saucepan sprayed lightly with non-stick cooking spray. Add chard to the pan and cook just until it is limp. Set it aside to cool.

5. Lightly coat a baking sheet with nonstick cooking spray.

6. Place a tortilla on the baking sheet.

Sprinkle shredded cheese evenly over the tortilla. Evenly spread the chard on top of the cheese. Cover the quesadilla with the remaining tortilla.

7. Lightly mist the top of the quesadilla with a bit more nonstick cooking spray. Bake in preheated oven for approximately 15 minutes.

8. Allow to cool and then cut into fourths. Transfer to the serving plate. Serve with low-fat sour cream, salsa, and/or guaca-mole, if desired. Enjoy!

Here are some ways to involve your children in cooking:

- Children can rinse the chard and cut it using child-sized knives or scissors, or they can tear it with their hands.

- With assistance, older children can hold the nonstick cooking spray 6 to 8 inches away from the pan and use a gentle sweeping motion to coat it. Younger children can place the tortillas on the sheet.

- Children can sprinkle the shredded cheese onto the tortillas and then top the cheese with a layer of chard.

- Remember to keep children away from sharp cutting utensils, electrical devices, and hot food and surfaces at all times!

Note: If you prefer a recipe that yields 6 entrée servings or 18 snack-sized portions, please ask for the classroom version.

Nutrition Information Per Serving

134 calories	6 g total fat
3 g saturated fat	13 g carbohydrates
2 g fiber	1 g sugar
15 mg cholesterol	250 mg sodium

Carrot Oatmeal Cookies

ESTIMATED TIME: 20 MINUTES
Yields 12 cookies

For this recipe, you will need these items:

INCLUDED IN THE RECIPE KIT:
¼ cup sugar
1 cup (3 ounces) shredded carrots,
    about 1½ medium-large carrots
1 cup white whole-wheat flour
½ cup rolled oats
½ teaspoon ground cinnamon
½ teaspoon baking powder
¼ teaspoon salt

FROM YOUR KITCHEN:
1 large egg
¼ cup canola or vegetable oil
½ teaspoon vanilla (optional)
Nonstick cooking spray or
    1-2 teaspoons vegetable oil

Prepare the recipe by following these steps:

1. Heat the oven to 375° F.

2. Spray a cookie sheet with nonstick cooking spray or lightly coat with vegetable oil.

3. Wash the carrots and grate them using a food processor or hand grater.

4. In a medium bowl, use a fork to beat the oil and sugar together until they're well combined.

5. In a small bowl, beat the egg using a fork. Add it to the oil mixture. Add the carrots.

6. In a large bowl, combine: flour, oats, cinnamon, baking powder, and salt. Stir until evenly combined.

7. Create a large well, or indentation, in the middle of the dry ingredients. Slowly add the oil mixture to it. Stir until the wet and dry ingredients are evenly combined.

8. Using a large dinner spoon, drop batter onto the cookie sheet, leaving a 2-inch space between the cookies.

9. Bake for 15 to 18 minutes or until golden brown.

10. Allow the cookies to cool before you serve them.

Here are some ways to involve your children in cooking:

❦ Children can help wash the carrots. If you're using a hand grater, you can hold the grater while children grate carrots, taking safety precautions to ensure children do not grate small pieces.

❦ Older children can measure the ingredients and younger children can pour the ingredients into the mixing bowls.

❦ Children can help scoop the cookie dough and drop it onto the baking sheets.

❦ Remember to keep children away from sharp cutting utensils, electrical devices, and hot food and surfaces at all times!

Nutrition Information Per Serving

120 calories	5 g total fat
< 1 g saturated fat	16 g carbohydrates
2 g fiber	4 g sugar
15 mg cholesterol	76 mg sodium

Butternut Squash Pancakes

ESTIMATED TIME: 30 MINUTES
Yields 4 servings

For this recipe, you will need these items:

INCLUDED IN THE RECIPE KIT:
¾ cup cooked butternut squash
½ cup white whole-wheat flour
½ teaspoon cinnamon
1 teaspoon brown sugar
¼ teaspoon salt
1 teaspoon baking powder

FROM YOUR KITCHEN:
1½ teaspoons canola or other
    vegetable oil
¾ cup milk
1 egg
Nonstick cooking spray
Optional: Maple syrup

Prepare the recipe by following these steps:

1. Scoop squash out of its skin and measure ¾ cup.

2. Place in a blender until well combined: squash, flour, cinnamon, brown sugar, salt, baking powder, canola oil, egg, and milk.

3. Lightly coat a griddle or large skillet with nonstick cooking spray.

4. Pour the batter onto griddle in silver-dollar-sized pancakes.

5. When the batter is fairly covered with bubbles, flip the pancakes. Cook until both sides are golden brown.

6. Allow the pancakes to cool and serve them with warm maple syrup, if desired.

Here are some ways to involve your children in cooking:

☙ Children can help scoop the squash out of its skin.

☙ Older children can measure the ingredients, and younger children can pour the ingredients into the blender

☙ Children can turn the blender on and off.

☙ Remember to keep children away from sharp cutting utensils, electrical devices, and hot food and surfaces at all times!

Note: If you prefer a recipe that yields 6 entrée servings or 18 snack-sized portions, please ask for the classroom version.

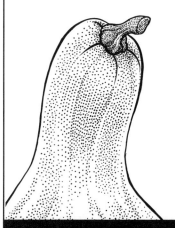

Nutrition Information Per Serving

140 calories	4 g total fat
1 g saturated fat	20 g carbohydrates
3.5 g fiber	4 g sugar
49 mg cholesterol	283 mg sodium

Pasta with Garlic-Parmesan Tomato Sauce

ESTIMATED TIME: 25 MINUTES
Yields 4 servings

For this recipe, you will need these items:

INCLUDED IN THE RECIPE KIT:
¼ pound whole-wheat pasta
1½ cups cherry tomatoes
1 clove fresh garlic
2 heaping tablespoons grated
    Parmesan cheese
2 tablespoons low-sodium
    vegetable broth

FROM YOUR KITCHEN:
1½ teaspoons olive or other
    vegetable oil

Prepare the recipe by following these steps:

1. Bring approximately 6 cups of water to a rolling boil over high heat.

2. Meanwhile, gently rinse the cherry tomatoes. Cut all of the tomatoes in half.

3. Remove the outer skin from the garlic. Crush the garlic clove in a garlic press, or use a knife to finely mince.

4. Add pasta to the boiling water and cook for approximately 10 minutes.

5. Add the tomatoes and broth to a blender. Use the pulse mechanism to coarsely chop and incorporate the ingredients.

6. When the pasta has finished cooking, remove from heat, drain, and rinse with cold water to stop it from cooking.

7. Heat the olive oil in a skillet on medium-high heat. When the oil is hot, add the minced garlic, cook for 30 seconds, and then add the tomato sauce from the blender. Reduce heat and simmer for about 5 minutes to cook off excess liquid.

8. Add the cooked pasta to the skillet and stir to coat it with the sauce. Heat for another minute or two, then remove from heat and transfer to a serving dish.

9. Sprinkle the cheese on top of the pasta.

Here are some suggested ways to involve your children in cooking:

❦ Children can rinse the cherry tomatoes and cut them in half using a child-sized knife.

❦ Children can scoop the halved tomatoes into the unplugged blender and measure and add the broth.

❦ Children can sprinkle the grated Parmesan cheese on top at the end of the recipe.

❦ Remember to keep children away from sharp cutting utensils, electrical devices, and hot food and surfaces at all times!

Nutrition Information Per Serving	
140 calories	3 g total fat
1 g saturated fat	24 g carbohydrates
3 g fiber	2 g sugar
0 mg cholesterol	75 mg sodium

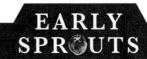

FAMILY RECIPE KIT

EARLY SPROUTS

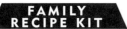

Green Bean Wontons with Dipping Sauce

ESTIMATED TIME: 30 MINUTES
Yields 4 servings

For this recipe, you will need these items:

INCLUDED IN THE RECIPE KIT:
1 cup green beans
8 wonton wrappers
2 tablespoons rice vinegar
1 tablespoon low-sodium, wheat-free
  tamari
1 teaspoon honey

FROM YOUR KITCHEN:
1 tablespoon canola or vegetable oil

Prepare the recipe by following these steps:

1. Clean the green beans and remove their stems. Shred the green beans using a food processor or chop them finely with a knife.

2. Heat the oil in a nonstick skillet over medium to high heat. Sauté the shredded green beans until they're tender. Allow them to cool.

3. To create a green bean wonton, take one wonton wrapper, place ½ tablespoon of shredded green beans in the center of the wrapper, wet all sides of the wonton with your finger, and then fold the wonton into a triangle. Press the edges together.

Repeat until you've made all 8 wontons, or as many of them as you want.

4. Heat a small amount of oil in the nonstick skillet.

5. Sauté the wontons 2 to 3 minutes per side or until slightly golden.

6. While the wontons are cooking, prepare the dipping sauce by mixing tamari, rice vinegar, and honey in a small bowl.

7. Remove the wontons from the pan. As soon as the wontons reach a safe eating temperature, serve with the dipping sauce.

Here are some ways to involve your children in cooking:

- Children can help wash the green beans, remove their stems, and snap the beans.

- Children may enjoy watching you process the green beans.

- Older children can measure, and younger children can pour ingredients into the mixing bowl. All ages can stir the ingredients.

- Children enjoy filling and folding their own wontons.

- Remember to keep children away from sharp cutting utensils, electrical devices, and hot food and surfaces at all times!

Note: If you prefer a recipe that yields 6 entrée servings or 18 snack-sized portions, please ask for the classroom version.

Nutrition Information Per Serving

45 calories	2 g total fat
0 g saturated fat	6 g carbohydrates
< 1 g fiber	1 g sugar
0 mg cholesterol	170 mg sodium

Confetti Corn Muffins

ESTIMATED TIME: 20 MINUTES, PLUS 20 MINUTES FOR BAKING
Yields 6 muffins or 12 mini muffins

For this recipe, you will need these items:

INCLUDED IN THE RECIPE KIT:
½ cup cornmeal (fine milled)
¼ cup white whole-wheat flour
½ teaspoon baking powder
¼ teaspoon baking soda
¾ cup low-fat plain yogurt
1½ tablespoons honey
⅓ cup shredded sharp cheddar cheese
¼ bell pepper

FROM YOUR KITCHEN:
⅛ teaspoon salt
1 large egg
Nonstick cooking spray or vegetable oil
1½ tablespoons canola or other vegetable oil

Prepare the recipe by following these steps:

1. Heat the oven to 400° F.

2. Coat the muffin tins well with nonstick cooking spray or wipe the tins with a paper towel coated with vegetable oil.

3. Clean the bell pepper and remove its seeds. Finely dice the pepper. Set the diced pepper aside.

4. Place in a large mixing bowl: cornmeal, flour, salt, baking powder, and baking soda (mixed in the bag that came in the kit).

5. Whisk together in a medium mixing bowl: yogurt, honey, eggs, and oil.

6. Create a well, or indentation, in the center of the dry mixture. Fill it with the wet ingredients. Gently stir until all the ingredients are incorporated. Do not overstir.

7. Gently fold half of the shredded cheddar cheese into the batter.

8. Fill the muffin tins three-quarters full. Sprinkle the diced bell peppers on top of the uncooked muffins, followed by the remaining cheddar cheese.

9. Bake 15 to 20 minutes or until golden brown. Allow to cool slightly before removing from pan. Enjoy!

Here are some ways to involve your children in cooking:

- Children can help wash, deseed, and chop peppers using a child-sized plastic knife. You can then chop the pepper more finely.

- Older children can measure, and younger children can pour ingredients into the mixing bowls. All ages can stir ingredients.

- Children can sprinkle the shredded cheese and bell pepper pieces on top of the muffins before baking.

- Remember to keep children away from sharp cutting utensils, electrical devices, and hot food and surfaces at all times!

Note: If you prefer a recipe that yields 6 entrée servings or 18 snack-sized portions, please ask for the classroom version.

Nutrition Information Per Serving (standard size muffin)

166 calories	7 g total fat
2 g saturated fat	20 g carbohydrates
2 g fiber	7 g sugar
40 mg cholesterol	200 mg sodium

Pita Pocket Pizzas

ESTIMATED TIME: 20 MINUTES
Yields 8 small servings

For this recipe, you will need these items:

INCLUDED IN THE RECIPE KIT:
4 to 6 Swiss chard leaves
4 tablespoons tomato sauce
1/8 teaspoon garlic powder and 1/8 teaspoon Italian spices (no salt added)
1/3 cup shredded mozzarella cheese
2 whole-wheat pita bread rounds

FROM YOUR KITCHEN:
2 teaspoons olive or other vegetable oil

Prepare the recipe by following these steps:

1. Heat the oven to 400° F.

2. Wash and dry the chard. Stack the washed chard leaves with all stems facing the same direction. Cut a triangle shape around the stems, separating the leaves from the stems. Stack the leaves again and chop finely.

3. Heat the oil in a skillet for about 1 minute. Then add chard and cook, stirring occasionally, for 2 minutes.

4. Remove the skillet from the heat. Carefully add the tomato sauce to pan, stirring gently until the leaves and sauce are combined.

5. Add the garlic powder and spices; stir.

6. Lay the pita bread on a large baking sheet.

7. Spread approximately 2 tablespoons of sauce on each pita round. Sprinkle cheese on top of each pita.

8. Bake for approximately 7 to 10 minutes or until the cheese is bubbly.

9. Remove from oven. Cut each round into 4 slices.

Here are some ways to involve your children in cooking:

- Children can help tear chard leaves into very small pieces for you to finely chop.

- Older children can measure the sauce and lay the pita bread on baking sheet.

- Have children spread the sauce on pita bread and then sprinkle the cheese on top.

- Remember to keep children away from sharp cutting utensils, electrical devices, and hot food and surfaces at all times!

Note: If you prefer a recipe that yields 6 entrée servings or 18 snack-sized portions, please ask for the classroom version.

Nutrition Information Per Serving

70 calories	2.5 g total fat
< 1 g saturated fat	10 g carbohydrates
2 g fiber	1 g sugar
5 mg cholesterol	220 mg sodium

Honey Glazed Carrots

ESTIMATED TIME: 40 TO 45 MINUTES
Yields 4 servings

For this recipe, you will need these items:

INCLUDED IN THE RECIPE KIT:
¾ pound carrots
1½ teaspoons low-sodium tamari
1 tablespoon butter
1½ tablespoons honey

Prepare the recipe by following these steps:

1. Wash and peel carrots.

2. Steam carrots until just tender. Rinse in a strainer under cold water to cool.

3. Cut carrots into bite size pieces.

4. Place butter and tamari in saucepan and cook over medium-low heat.

5. Once the butter is melted, add the honey.

6. Stir in steamed carrots and mix until all carrots are glazed.

Here are some ways to involve your children in cooking:

🌱 Children can wash the carrots. Once carrots are steamed (and cooled), encourage children to cut each into bite-size pieces with a child-safe knife.

🌱 Remember to keep sharp cutting utensils, electrical devices, and hot food and surfaces away from children at all times!

Note: If you prefer a recipe that yields 6 entrée servings or 18 snack-sized portions, please ask for the classroom version.

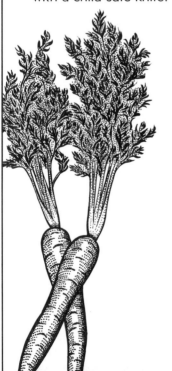

Nutrition Information Per Serving

65 calories	2.5 g total fat
1.5 g saturated fat	11 g carbohydrates
2 g fiber	8 g sugar
6 mg cholesterol	159 mg sodium

Banana Squash Smoothie

ESTIMATED TIME: 10 MINUTES
Yields 4 servings

For this recipe, you will need these items:

INCLUDED IN THE RECIPE KIT:
1 cup butternut squash, cooked
1 cup low-fat vanilla yogurt
1 banana

FROM YOUR KITCHEN:
2 cups low-fat milk
1 teaspoon vanilla

Prepare the recipe by following these steps:

1. Cut squash in half lengthwise, leaving seeds in, and bake until the squash is tender.

2. Scoop the seeds out of the squash and discard them.

3. Scoop the squash out of its skin and measure 1 cup.

4. Combine all the ingredients in the blender and blend until smooth. Enjoy!

Here are some ways to involve your children in cooking:

- Children can help remove the seeds from the cooled squash by gently scraping the seeds out with spoons and can peel the banana.

- Children can measure the ingredients into the blender or into a separate container.

- It may be fun for children to push the buttons on the blender!

- Remember to keep children away from electric cords and blender blades.

Note: If you prefer a recipe that yields 6 entrée servings or 18 snack-sized portions, please ask for the classroom version.

Nutrition Information Per Serving

167 calories	3 g total fat
2 g saturated fat	28 g carbohydrates
3 g fiber	20 g sugar
13 mg cholesterol	90 mg sodium

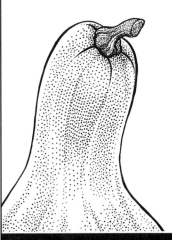

FAMILY RECIPE KIT

EARLY SPROUTS

English Muffin Pizzas with Homemade Sauce

ESTIMATED TIME: 20 MINUTES, PLUS 15 MINUTES BAKING TIME
Yields 4 servings

For this recipe, you will need these items:

INCLUDED IN THE RECIPE KIT:
1 cup cherry tomatoes, washed (about 10 tomatoes)
2 whole wheat English muffins
¾ cup shredded part-skim mozzarella cheese

FROM YOUR KITCHEN:
½ teaspoon sugar
1½ teaspoons olive or other vegetable oil

Prepare the recipe by following these steps:

1. Heat the oven to 400° F.

2. Rinse the cherry tomatoes and cut them in half.

3. Heat 1½ teaspoons oil in the skillet over medium heat. Add the halved tomatoes to the skillet; sprinkle them with the sugar. Sauté for about 5 to 6 minutes.

4. Transfer the contents of the skillet to a blender or food processor and purée. Pour the puréed tomato sauce into a shallow bowl.

5. Split the English muffins in half and place them on an ungreased baking sheet.

6. To assemble each pizza, spoon about 2 tablespoons of sauce onto English muffin "crusts," spreading it with back of a spoon. Cover each pizza with a handful of cheese.

7. Bake the pizzas in oven for about 10 to 15 minutes or until the cheese is bubbly and just beginning to brown.

8. Allow the pizzas to cool slightly and cut them in halves or quarters. Transfer to a serving platter, serve, and enjoy!

Here are some ways to involve your children in cooking:

- Children can rinse the cherry tomatoes. They can practice cutting the tomatoes in half on a plate or cutting board, using child-sized plastic knives.

- Children can assemble the English muffin pizzas by spreading the sauce and sprinkling the cheese on top. Assist as needed.

- Remember to keep children away from sharp cutting utensils, electrical devices, and hot food and surfaces at all times!

Note: If you prefer a recipe that yields 6 entrée servings or 18 snack-sized portions, please ask for the classroom version.

Nutrition Information Per Serving

140 calories	6 g total fat
2.5 g saturated fat	16 g carbohydrates
3 g fiber	4 g sugar
14 mg cholesterol	289 mg sodium

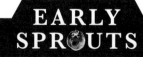

FAMILY RECIPE KIT

EARLY SPROUTS

Sesame Seed Green Beans

ESTIMATED TIME: 30 MINUTES
Yields 4 servings

For this recipe, you will need these items:

INCLUDED IN THE RECIPE KIT:
⅓ to ½ pound fresh green beans
2 tablespoons sesame seeds for sprinkling

FROM YOUR KITCHEN:
Salt and pepper to taste
1 teaspoon olive oil

Prepare the recipe by following these steps:

1. Wash the green beans and trim off their ends. Snap the beans in half.

2. Pour the oil into a skillet and warm it over medium heat.

3. Add the green beans to skillet and sauté them 5 to 8 minutes or until tender.

4. Season the beans with salt and pepper.

5. Serve the beans in small bowls and enjoy! Invite your family to sprinkle sesame seeds on their green beans if they like.

Here are some ways to involve your children in cooking:

🌱 Children can wash the beans, snap off their stems, and snap the beans in half.

🌱 Children can season the cooked beans with salt and pepper and sprinkle sesame seeds on their beans, if they choose.

🌱 Remember to keep children away from sharp cutting utensils, electrical devices, and hot food and surfaces at all times!

Note: If you prefer a recipe that yields 6 entrée servings or 18 snack-sized portions, please ask for the classroom version.

Nutrition Information Per Serving

40 calories	2.5 g total fat
0 g saturated fat	4 g carbohydrates
2 g fiber	1 g sugar
0 mg cholesterol	0 mg sodium

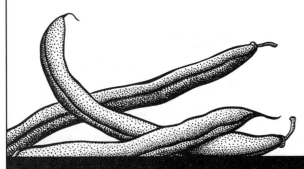

FAMILY RECIPE KIT

EARLY SPROUTS

Bell Pepper Veggie Burgers

ESTIMATED TIME: 25 MINUTES, PLUS 10 MINUTES BAKING TIME
Yields 4 servings

For this recipe, you will need these items:

INCLUDED IN THE RECIPE KIT:
7½ ounces canned low-sodium black
    beans (half of a 15-ounce can)
⅓ cup Italian bread crumbs
⅓ large red bell pepper
¼ cup shredded cheddar cheese
2 small or 1 large whole wheat pita
    pockets

FROM YOUR KITCHEN:
1 teaspoon vegetable oil
1 egg
Ketchup for serving
Nonstick cooking spray

Prepare the recipe by following these steps:

1. Heat the oven to broil.* Spray a baking sheet generously with nonstick cooking spray.

2. Wash the bell pepper and remove its stem and seeds. Cut the pepper into small pieces.

3. Place 1 teaspoon of vegetable oil in a small skillet. Heat the oil over medium heat and add the pepper pieces. Sauté.

4. In a small bowl, beat the egg lightly with a fork.

5. Drain and rinse black beans with cool water. Place the beans in large bowl and mash well with a potato masher or large fork.

6. Add bread crumbs, lightly beaten egg, and cheese. Stir until the ingredients are evenly combined.

7. Form the burger mixture into 4 small patties and place them on the baking sheet. Place the sheet in the oven 4 to 6 inches from the flame. Broil for 5 minutes, flip the burgers, and broil an additional 5 to 6 minutes. Watch closely to prevent burning.

8. When the burgers are done, allow them to cool slightly before placing them in halved or quartered pita pockets. Serve with plenty of ketchup and enjoy!

Stovetop Alternative: Burgers can also be cooked on the stovetop in a skillet with a small amount of vegetable oil. Cook over medium high heat for 5 minutes on each side.

Here are some ways to involve your children in cooking:

❦ Children can rinse the bell pepper and remove its seeds.

❦ Children can dump and rinse the beans, and then help mash the beans, assist with breaking and scrambling eggs, measure the ingredients, and help mix.

❦ Children can form mixture into small patties and place them on the baking sheet.

❦ Using a child-sized knife, children can cut pita pockets in halves or quarters to create the burger buns.

❦ Remember to keep children away from sharp cutting utensils, electrical devices, and hot food and surfaces at all times!

Nutrition Information Per Serving (1 burger + 1 tsp. ketchup)

170 calories	6 g total fat
2 g saturated fat	26 g carbohydrates
5 g fiber	4 g sugar
50 mg cholesterol	500 mg sodium

FAMILY RECIPE KIT

EARLY SPROUTS

Lemony Swiss Chard Pasta

ESTIMATED TIME: 40 MINUTES
Yields 4 servings

For this recipe, you will need these items:

INCLUDED IN THE RECIPE KIT:
1/3 pound whole-wheat pasta
3 leaves of Swiss chard
1/2 small or medium lemon
5 ounces of feta cheese

FROM YOUR KITCHEN:
Pinch of sea salt and pepper
2 teaspoons olive oil or other
vegetable oil

Prepare the recipe by following these steps:

1. Bring a pot of water to a boil. Add pasta to the pot and cook for 10 minutes or until *al dente*, stirring occasionally.

2. Meanwhile, wash the chard, remove its stems, and cut the chard into small, 1/3- to 1/2-inch pieces.

3. Squeeze the lemon juice into a large bowl.

4. In the large bowl, whisk together the lemon juice, salt, pepper, and olive oil.

5. Chop the feta cheese into small pieces.

6. When pasta is cooked, add the pasta, chard, and feta to the bowl of dressing.

7. Toss until well combined.

Here are some ways to involve your children in cooking:

- Invite children to help wash the chard. Using child-sized knives or kitchen scissors, children cut the chard and feta into small pieces.

- Cut the lemon into small wedges and invite children to help squeeze the lemon juice into a large bowl and whisk the dressing together.

- Children can help measure and pour the dressing ingredients.

- Children enjoy helping stir the pasta salad together until well combined.

- Remember to keep children away from sharp cutting utensils, electrical devices, and hot food and surfaces at all times!

Note: If you prefer a recipe that yields 6 entrée servings or 18 snack-sized portions, please ask for the classroom version.

Nutrition Information Per Serving

210 calories	7 g total fat
3 g saturated fat	32 g carbohydrates
4 g fiber	1 g sugar
15 mg cholesterol	350 mg sodium

EARLY SPROUTS

Carrot Sticks with Vanilla Dip

ESTIMATED TIME: 15 MINUTES
Yields 4 servings

For this recipe, you will need these items:

INCLUDED IN THE RECIPE KIT:
20 to 25 baby carrots
½ cup vanilla low-fat yogurt
¼ teaspoon cinnamon
1½ teaspoons honey

Prepare the recipe by following these steps:

1. Measure the yogurt, honey, and cinnamon into a small bowl.

2. Mix together and serve it as a dip with the carrots.

Here are some ways to involve your children in cooking:

❦ Children can wash the carrots.

❦ Children can help measure and mix the ingredients in the dip.

Note: If you prefer a recipe that yields 6 entrée servings or 18 snack-sized portions, please ask for the classroom version.

Nutrition Information Per Serving

35 calories	0 g total fat
0 g saturated fat	7 g carbohydrates
< 1 g fiber	6 g sugar
0 mg cholesterol	40 mg sodium

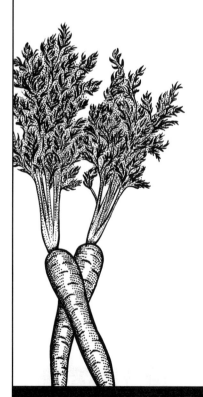

Butternut Squash Muffins

ESTIMATED TIME: 20 MINUTES, PLUS 20 TO 25 MINUTES BAKING TIME
Yields 6 muffins or 12 mini muffins

For this recipe, you will need these items:

INCLUDED IN THE RECIPE KIT:
1 cup grated butternut squash
1 cup white whole wheat flour
1½ tablespoons pure maple syrup
2 tablespoons brown sugar, packed
½ teaspoon cinnamon
1 teaspoon baking powder
¼ teaspoon salt

FROM YOUR KITCHEN:
2 tablespoons canola or other
    vegetable oil
1 egg or two egg whites
½ cup low-fat milk

Prepare the recipe by following these steps:

1. Heat the oven to 350° F.

2. Prepare muffin cups with paper baking cups or nonstick cooking spray.

3. In a medium bowl, stir together grated squash, brown sugar, and maple syrup. Let sit for 10 minutes.

4. In a larger bowl, combine flour, baking powder, and salt.

5. Add squash mixture to flour mixture. Add the remaining ingredients and stir until flour mixture is fully moistened: milk, egg, and canola oil. Do not overmix.

6. Spoon batter into prepared muffin cups until about two-thirds full.

7. Bake muffins for 20 to 25 minutes or until a toothpick inserted into the center of a muffin comes out clean.

Here are some ways to involve your children in cooking:

❦ While the oven is preheating, have children spray the muffin pan lightly.

❦ Children can help measure and pour the ingredients into bowls.

❦ After the ingredients are measured, children can mix them together, being careful not to overmix lest batter become tough.

❦ At a safe distance from the oven, allow children to observe while an adult places the muffin pan in the oven. Allow children to watch the rising muffins, if it can be done safely.

❦ Remember to keep children away from sharp cutting utensils, electrical devices, and hot food and surfaces at all times!

Note: If you prefer a recipe that yields 6 entrée servings or 18 snack-sized portions, please ask for the classroom version.

Nutrition Information Per Serving (standard size muffin)

190 calories	6 g total fat
1 g saturated fat	30 g carbohydrates
4 g fiber	9 g sugar
30 mg cholesterol	180 mg sodium

Tomato and Cheese Quesadillas

ESTIMATED TIME: 20 MINUTES, PLUS 15 MINUTES BAKING TIME
Yields 4 servings

For this recipe, you will need these items:

INCLUDED IN THE RECIPE KIT:
1 medium tomato
2/3 cup shredded Monterey Jack cheese
2 whole-wheat tortillas or wraps

FROM YOUR KITCHEN:
Nonstick cooking spray
Optional: salsa, low-fat sour cream,
    and/or guacamole

Prepare the recipe by following these steps:

1. Heat the oven to 400° F.

2. Wash the tomato and cut it into thick slices.

3. Lightly coat a baking sheet with nonstick cooking spray.

4. Place a tortilla on the baking sheet. Sprinkle the shredded cheese evenly over the tortilla. Top the cheese with a single layer of tomato slices. Cover the quesadilla with the remaining tortilla.

5. Lightly mist the top of each quesadilla with a bit more vegetable oil spray. Bake in the oven for approximately 15 minutes.

6. Allow the quesadilla to cool and then cut it into fourths. Transfer to a serving plate. Serve with salsa, low-fat sour cream, and/ or guacamole, if desired. Enjoy!

Here are some ways to involve your children in cooking:

- Children can rinse the tomato in the sink. Have them practice cutting the tomato, using a child-sized knife and working over a small plate.

- Invite children to sprinkle the shredded cheese onto the tortilla. Demonstrate, and then encourage them to top the cheese with a layer of tomato slices.

- Show older children how to hold the nonstick cooking spray 6 to 8 inches away from the pan and use a gentle sweeping motion to coat it. Younger children may place the tortilla on the sheets.

- Remember to keep children away from sharp cutting utensils, electrical devices, and hot food and surfaces at all times!

Note: If you prefer a recipe that yields 6 entrée servings or 18 snack-sized portions, please ask for the classroom version.

Nutrition Information Per Serving

130 calories	6 g total fat
2.5 g saturated fat	13 g carbohydrates
1 g fiber	2 g sugar
15 mg cholesterol	160 mg sodium

Green and Orange Pasta Salad

ESTIMATED TIME: 20 TO 25 MINUTES,
PLUS AN OPTIONAL 30 MINUTES OF REFRIGERATOR TIME TO COOL
Yields 6 servings

For this recipe, you will need these items:

INCLUDED IN THE RECIPE KIT:
1 tablespoon balsamic vinegar
1½ tablespoons olive oil
½ pound whole wheat pasta
½ pound green beans
3 carrots
½ cup shredded Parmesan cheese

FROM YOUR KITCHEN:
Salt and pepper to taste

Prepare the recipe by following these steps:

1. Bring a pot of water to boil for the pasta.

2. Wash green beans and snap off stems.

3. Cut or break the green beans into bite-sized pieces and place them in a steamer or a skillet filled with ¾ inch of water.

4. Steam or cook the green beans over high heat for 5 to 8 minutes or until tender. Cool the beans by rinsing them under cold water.

5. Wash and peel the carrots.

6. Shred the carrots in a food processor or dice them.

7. When the water is boiling, add the pasta and cook for 10 minutes or until *al dente*. When the pasta is done, drain it in a strainer. Rinse the strainer of pasta under cold water.

8. In a large bowl, combine vinegar, oil, cheese, salt, and pepper. Add pasta, carrots, and green beans. Mix until combined.

9. Serve immediately or store in a refrigerator for 30 minutes to cool.

Note: If you're planning to eat the pasta salad several hours later, please wait to add vinegar and oil until just before serving. Otherwise the pasta will absorb all of the dressing.

Here are some ways to involve your children in cooking:

❦ Children can wash the green beans, snap off their stems, and cut or snap them into small pieces.

❦ Children can help wash carrots and enjoy watching you process them.

❦ Older children can measure ingredients and younger children can pour ingredients.

❦ Remember to keep children away from sharp cutting utensils, electrical devices, and hot food and surfaces at all times!

Nutrition Information Per Serving

220 calories	6 g total fat
2 g saturated fat	35 g carbohydrates
5 g fiber	3 g sugar
5 mg cholesterol	150 mg sodium

Bell Pepper and Pineapple Fried Rice
ESTIMATED TIME: 20 MINUTES, PLUS TIME TO COOK THE RICE
Yields 4 servings

For this recipe, you will need these items:

INCLUDED IN THE RECIPE KIT:
2/3 cup brown or basmati rice
1 fresh bell pepper, washed
1 clove fresh garlic (to yield about
    1/2 teaspoon crushed)
1 small piece fresh ginger root (about
    1 teaspoon grated)
1/4 cup canned crushed pineapple (in its
    own juice)
1 tablespoon low-sodium, wheat-free
    tamari

FROM YOUR KITCHEN:
2 tablespoons vegetable oil

Prepare the recipe by following these steps:

1. Ahead of time, cook rice.

2. Rinse the brown rice under running water in a strainer and place the rice in a pot with 1 1/3 cups water.

3. Bring to a boil. Then lower heat and simmer, covered, for 25 minutes or until all the water is absorbed and the rice is tender. You may need to add a little more water.

4. Remove the pot from the stove and let it sit, covered, for 5 minutes.

5. Wash, deseed, and finely chop the bell pepper.

6. Peel and finely grate the ginger using a cheese grater, or finely dice it.

7. Remove the outer skin from the garlic, crush it in a garlic press, or finely chop it.

8. Add to a skillet or wok: oil, pepper, ginger, and garlic. Raise the heat to medium-high and sauté until the peppers are soft. Add rice and pineapple.

9. Gently stir the mixture to disperse the oil and flavorings. Add the tamari and heat for an additional 1 to 2 minutes.

10. Remove from the heat, and allow the mixture to cool slightly. Transfer to a serving platter. Serve family style and enjoy!

Here are some ways to involve your children in cooking:

☀ Children can help wash, deseed, and finely chop the pepper.

☀ Children can remove outer skin from garlic.

☀ Remember to keep children away from sharp cutting utensils, electrical devices, and hot food and surfaces at all times!

Nutrition Information Per Serving

193 calories	8 g total fat
1 g saturated fat	28 g carbohydrates
2 g fiber	3 g sugar
0 mg cholesterol	250 mg sodium

FAMILY RECIPE KIT

EARLY SPROUTS

Cheesy Swiss Chard Squares

ESTIMATED TIME: 30 MINUTES PLUS 25 TO 30 MINUTES FOR BAKING
Yields 4 servings

For this recipe, you will need these items:

INCLUDED IN THE RECIPE KIT:
2 slices whole wheat bread
½ bunch Swiss chard
¼ cup grated Parmesan cheese
¼ cup mozzarella cheese

FROM YOUR KITCHEN:
1 teaspoon canola or other
    vegetable oil
2 eggs
Salt and pepper to taste
Nonstick cooking spray

Prepare the recipe by following these steps:

1. Heat the oven to 350° F.

2. Toast the bread in a toaster. Allow the slices to cool, then chop or tear them into very small cubes.

3. Wash the chard, remove its stems, and chop or tear it into small pieces.

4. Cook chard in 1 teaspoon oil in a covered skillet over medium heat for 4 to 5 minutes. Drain any excess liquid.

5. Whisk eggs in a large mixing bowl.

6. Add and stir until well-combined: chard, bread, cheese, salt, and pepper.

7. Lightly coat a casserole dish or 8-inch by 8-inch cake pan with nonstick cooking spray.

8. Place the mixture in the prepared pan.

9. Bake for 25 to 30 minutes. Cool and then cut into small squares.

10. Serve and enjoy.

Here are some ways to involve your children in cooking:

❦ After toasting the bread, invite children to help cut or tear the slices into very small pieces.

❦ Invite children to help wash the chard, remove its stems, and cut it into small pieces.

❦ Older children can measure ingredients, and younger children can pour ingredients into the mixing bowl.

❦ Children can stir the mixture.

❦ Children can help pour the ingredients from the mixing bowl into the casserole dish.

❦ Remember to keep children away from sharp cutting utensils, electrical devices, and hot food and surfaces at all times!

Note: If you prefer a recipe that yields 6 entrée servings or 18 snack-sized portions, please ask for the classroom version.

Nutrition Information Per Serving

123 calories	7 g total fat
2.5 g saturated fat	9 g carbohydrates
1 g fiber	2 g sugar
95 mg cholesterol	300 mg sodium

FAMILY RECIPE KIT

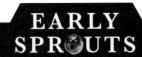

EARLY SPROUTS

Carrot Muffins

ESTIMATED TIME: 20 MINUTES, PLUS 20 MINUTES BAKING TIME
Yields 6 muffins or 12 mini muffins

For this recipe, you will need these items:

INCLUDED IN THE RECIPE KIT:
¾ cup white whole-wheat flour
½ teaspoon baking powder
½ teaspoon baking soda
1 teaspoon ground cinnamon
½ cup shredded carrots
⅓ cup maple syrup
2 tablespoons orange juice
¼ cup golden raisins
2½ tablespoons canola oil

FROM YOUR KITCHEN:
1 large egg
Nonstick cooking spray
¼ teaspoon salt

Prepare the recipe by following these steps:

1. Heat the oven to 400° F.

2. Lightly grease a standard 6-muffin pan, a mini muffin pan, or an 8-inch by 8-inch cake pan with nonstick cooking spray.

3. In a medium bowl, whisk together the eggs and maple syrup.

4. Stir in shredded carrots, orange juice, golden raisins, and vegetable oil.

5. In a large bowl, combine flour, baking powder, baking soda, cinnamon, and salt.

6. Create a well, or indentation, in the middle of the dry ingredients. Slowly pour the liquid ingredients into the well. Mix just until the dry ingredients are moistened. Do not overmix, or the muffins will be tough.

7. Divide the muffin batter into the muffin cups or pour into the cake pan. Bake for approximately 20 minutes or until a toothpick inserted into the center of a muffin comes out clean. (Mini muffins bake much faster than regular muffins.) Cool and serve.

Here are some ways to involve your children in cooking:

❦ Children may enjoy watching you shred the carrots. They can push the food processor's *on* button.

❦ Older children can measure ingredients, and younger children can pour ingredients. Children can stir ingredients together.

❦ Children enjoy cracking eggs and spooning the final mixture into the muffin cups.

❦ Remember to keep children away from sharp cutting utensils, electrical devices, and hot food and surfaces at all times!

Note: If you prefer a recipe that yields 6 entrée servings or 18 snack-sized portions, please ask for the classroom version.

Nutrition Information Per Serving (standard size muffin)

200 calories	7 g total fat
< 1 g saturated fat	31 g carbohydrates
3 g fiber	16 g sugar
30 mg cholesterol	250 mg sodium

Butternut Squash Fries

ESTIMATED TIME: 30 MINUTES, PLUS 20 MINUTES BAKING TIME
Yields 6 servings

For this recipe, you will need these items:

INCLUDED IN THE RECIPE KIT:
½ medium butternut squash

FROM YOUR KITCHEN:
Salt
Nonstick cooking spray

Prepare the recipe by following these steps:

1. Heat the oven to 425° F.

2. Place the squash cut-side down in a baking dish with about half an inch of water. Bake for 20 to 25 minutes, frequently checking for tenderness. Do not overcook the squash.

3. Allow the squash to cool.

4. Deseed and scoop out squash in large chunks.

5. Cut the baked squash chunks into french-fry shapes.

6. Spray a baking sheet with nonstick cooking spray.

7. Place the fries on the baking sheet. Sprinkle them lightly with salt.

8. Place the tray in oven and bake for approximately 20 minutes, turning the fries over halfway through baking process. The fries are done when they start to brown on the edges and get crispy.

9. Serve alone or with favorite condiment or dip.

Here are some ways to involve your children in cooking:

- Children can help spray the nonstick cooking spray onto the baking sheet.

- Show children how they can help remove the remaining seeds from the squash by using a spoon to gently scrape them onto a plate or into a garbage container.

- Guide children in cutting the squash into french-fry-shaped pieces using a child-sized knife. Have children gently lay the fries on the baking sheet.

- At a safe distance from the oven, allow children to look at the fries when they are done so they can distinguish the brown and crispy-looking ones from the slightly cooked fries. Remind them of how the fries looked before baking.

- Remember to keep children away from sharp cutting utensils, electrical devices, and hot food and surfaces at all times!

Note: If you prefer a recipe that yields 6 entrée servings or 18 snack-sized portions, please ask for the classroom version.

Nutrition Information Per Serving

64 calories	0 g total fat
0 g saturated fat	17 g carbohydrates
3 g fiber	3 g sugar
0 mg cholesterol	151 mg sodium

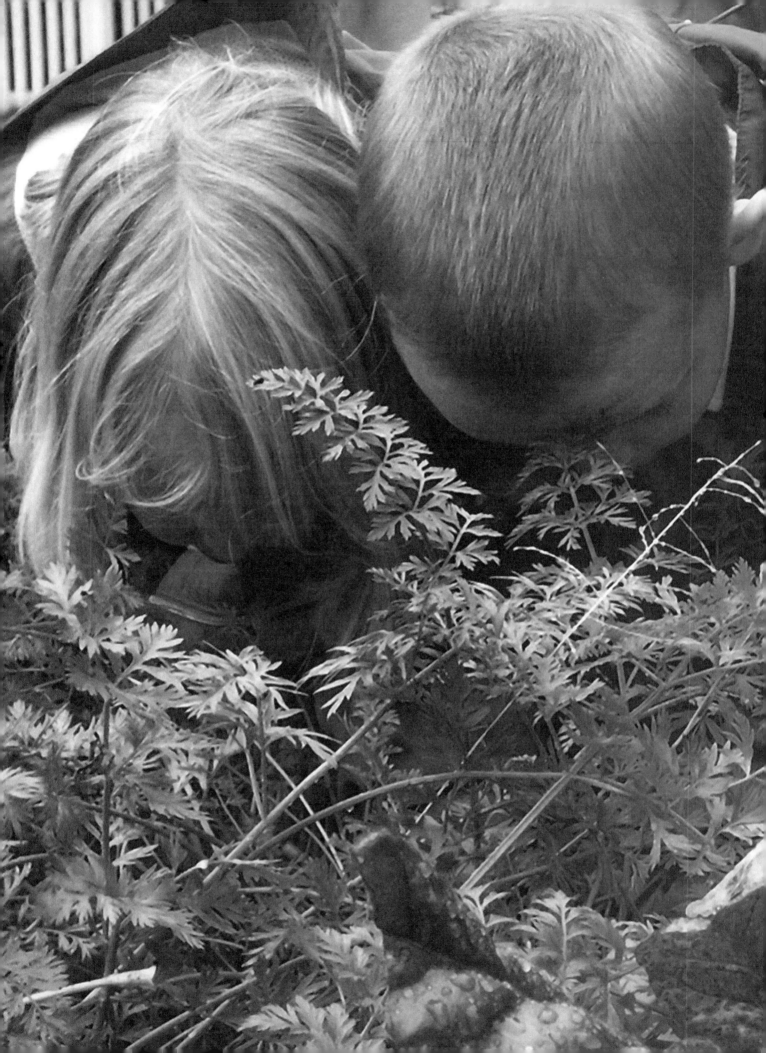

Part 3

SHARING
the
HARVEST

THIRTEEN

WHAT WE HAVE LEARNED
Research Process and Results

As you know, Early Sprouts is a research-based program, but implementing Early Sprouts does not require that you conduct research. In this age of research-based curriculum, you can rest assured knowing we are conducting the ongoing research that demonstrates the success of this program. Our research provides you with the confidence that this is a quality program for improving the eating habits of young children. We implement our research during the program and use several methods to share what we have learned from children, teachers, and families.

The Early Sprouts program was designed to apply knowledge gained from previous research studies that focused on children's food preferences and techniques of behavioral change. As part of our work, we want to share information with others about preschool children and their willingness to eat vegetables. To accomplish this goal, we are studying how the Early Sprouts approach affects the eating preferences and habits of children and their families. We have been collecting two types of information—numerical (quantitative) and verbal (qualitative). The numerical, or quantitative, information measures two things: children's willingness to taste and children's preference for the six target vegetables and novel vegetables, such as beets, summer squash, and cauliflower. We use these data to compile and analyze statistics that scientifically support the impact of our program. Equally important is the time we have spent collecting the words of those participating in the program. We collect written feedback, document our observations of children through anecdotal records, and conduct interviews with children, families, and teachers about their experiences with the program. We digest their written and verbal feedback and come up with themes that help us take a qualitative look at what we have accomplished.

Effective research is usually guided by carefully developed research questions that build on prior knowledge. Our research questions focus on children's vegetable consumption and on family behaviors.

- ☙ Will children participating in the Early Sprouts curriculum respond more favorably to specific vegetables over time?
- ☙ Will preschoolers be more willing to taste new foods after participating in the program?
- ☙ Will families make any changes in their food habits as a result of participating in Early Sprouts?

We gather data at different times of the year and in different ways. Here are the research strategies we use with each of the audiences involved in the project: children, teachers, families.

Tools for Gathering Information from Children

Children's preference for a particular food is the strongest predictor of their consumption of that food (Birch 1979, Morris and Zidenberg-Cherr 2002)—in other words, children eat more of foods they prefer and less of foods they think they don't like. To assess the impact of the program on children's eating habits, we use a variety of methods to gather information. Informal methods include observation, anecdotal records, photo documentation, teacher interviews, and family reports. We use taste testing as a more formal assessment of children's interest in vegetables. To measure children's taste preferences for vegetables, we use a child-friendly vegetable game. We provide each child with an individual sample of the specific vegetables we are testing. To play the game, we invite each child to choose and taste the vegetables, one vegetable at a time. Children are measured individually to avoid being influenced by other children. They are allowed to say "no thanks" to individual vegetables and are not required to taste all of the vegetables in one sitting. When we describe how to play the game, we show the children three faces and describe them this way:

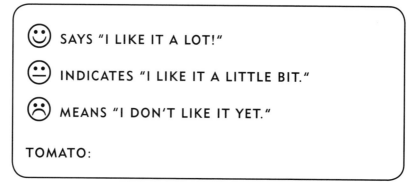

☺ SAYS "I LIKE IT A LOT!"

😐 INDICATES "I LIKE IT A LITTLE BIT."

☹ MEANS "I DON'T LIKE IT YET."

TOMATO:

These descriptive phrases are very important. The way we use language influences how we think and feel. By describing the frowning face as "I don't like it yet," we are communicating that not liking the food is an acceptable response. We are also suggesting that at some time in the future children may find they do like the food "a little bit" or maybe even "a lot." We intentionally do not label the smiling face the "yummy" face or the frowning one the "yucky" face. We want to avoid stereotypical judgments about food and confusion between foods we don't like and dirty or poisonous substances. Negative judgments are difficult to change, especially when they are influenced by social norms or powerful people. Remember that children at this age are very influenced by those around them. Our tone of voice, facial expressions, and words all need to be positive. We want to allow children to decide independently what they think about a particular vegetable. We want to leave open the possibility for development and change.

After tasting or handling each vegetable, we ask children which face describes their reaction to the vegetable. We record their willingness to taste and their response to each vegetable. Children are also invited to taste novel vegetables not included in the program. By including different vegetables in the taste-preference testing, we learn if the program helps children become more adventurous in their willingness to try new foods. Taste-preference testing occurs at the beginning, middle, and end of the program to assess change over time.

Faces Used in the Preference Test

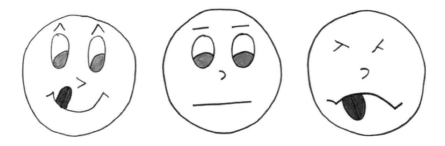

TASTE: YES   NO

Note: Hedonic face scale developed by Leann Birch at Pennsylvania State University. The tool has been adapted for use with the Early Sprouts program.

Tools for Gathering Information from Teachers

Regular feedback meetings between teachers and the research team provide opportunities for dialogue, troubleshooting, and ongoing feedback. In fact, information from teachers is regularly used to modify and improve the curriculum. The pacing of the program, which focuses on one vegetable each week, came from teachers. Sensory activities were revised to be made more developmentally appropriate, include both gross- and fine-motor skills, and involve both garden- and classroom-based experiences. Recipes have been added, subtracted, and modified based on what actually happened in the classroom. Teachers have identified many ways in which the curriculum helps meet other learning goals for young children. The curriculum we present in this book is a direct result of feedback from the classrooms and teachers involved and merges knowledge and application of child nutrition and child development.

Tools for Gathering Information from Families

We collect information from families at the beginning and at the end of the twenty-four-week curriculum, as well as every time a Family Recipe Kit goes home. Using a structured survey, we personally interview an adult member of each family at the start and finish of the Early Sprouts curriculum. The interviewer records the answer to each question on a printed form. The survey includes vegetable consumption patterns and the availability of vegetables and fruits (canned, fresh, frozen, dried) in the home at the time of the survey. We read a list of vegetables and ask the family member to identify: 1) if their child ate the vegetable during the past week and 2) how frequently it was eaten. We also ask families what other vegetables and fruits are available in the home. (You will find a sample of the Food Frequency Questionnaire below and a sample of the Food Availability Interview Questions on page 174.)

FOOD FREQUENCY QUESTIONNAIRE

FOOD ITEM	DURING THIS PAST WEEK, DID YOUR CHILD EAT THE FOLLOWING FOOD ITEM? (YES OR NO)	IF YES, ENTER THE NUMBER OF TIMES PER WEEK OR PER DAY (W OR D)
1. Asparagus	Yes or No	W or D
2. Artichoke	Yes or No	W or D
3. Avocado	Yes or No	W or D
4. Beets	Yes or No	W or D
5. Bell or other pepper	Yes or No	W or D
6. Broccoli	Yes or No	W or D
7. Beans (chickpea, pinto, black, lima, refried, etc.) or bean soup	Yes or No	W or D
8. Brussels sprout	Yes or No	W or D
9. Cabbage	Yes or No	W or D
10. Carrots	Yes or No	W or D

11. Cauliflower	Yes *or* No		W *or* D
12. Celery	Yes *or* No		W *or* D
13. Corn	Yes *or* No		W *or* D
14. Cucumber	Yes *or* No		W *or* D
15. Eggplant	Yes *or* No		W *or* D
16. Green, wax, or string bean	Yes *or* No		W *or* D
17. Lettuce/salad greens	Yes *or* No		W *or* D
18. Baked, boiled, or mashed potato	Yes *or* No		W *or* D
19. French fries	Yes *or* No		W *or* D
20. Sweet potatoes or yam	Yes *or* No		W *or* D
21. Radish	Yes *or* No		W *or* D
22. Pea or sugar snap pea	Yes *or* No		W *or* D
23. Spinach	Yes *or* No		W *or* D
24. Swiss chard	Yes *or* No		W *or* D
25. Kale, collard, or other dark leafy green	Yes *or* No		W *or* D
26. Tomatoes	Yes *or* No		W *or* D
27. Butternut squash	Yes *or* No		W *or* D
28. Acorn, pumpkin, or other winter squash	Yes *or* No		W *or* D
29. Zucchini or other summer squash	Yes *or* No		W *or* D
30. Okra	Yes *or* No		W *or* D
31. Turnip/parsnip	Yes *or* No		W *or* D
32. Other:_____	Yes *or* No		W *or* D
33. Other:_____	Yes *or* No		W *or* D
34. Other:_____	Yes *or* No		W *or* D

We are interested in any differences in the consumption of vegetables by the child in the home during the course of the twenty-four weeks. The information gathered from families helps us determine if any change is occurring in the foods available in the home. If the child is eating more vegetables and more vegetables are available, we assume that vegetables are being served more frequently at home. We tally the responses and compare the information reported at the beginning of the program with the answers collected after week 24.

INTERVIEW QUESTIONS ABOUT FOOD AVAILABILITY

Please tell me what fruits and vegetables your currently have in your home:

1. What canned vegetables, if any, do you currently have in your home?
2. What frozen vegetables, if any, do you currently have in your home?
3. What fresh vegetables, if any, do you currently have in your home?
4. What dried vegetables (beans, sun-dried tomatoes, etc.), if any, do you currently have in your home?
5. What canned fruits, if any, do you currently have in your home?
6. What frozen fruits, if any, do you currently have in your home?
7. What fresh fruits, if any, do you currently have in your home?
8. What dried fruits, if any, do you currently have in your home?

Families also provide regular feedback on the Family Recipe Kits by completing a brief questionnaire. (You have already seen a sample of this questionnaire included in chapter 12.) We tally the responses to determine which recipes are most popular at home. This allows us to analyze mathematically the amount of family participation with the Family Recipe Kits. From this information, we can determine the number of additional exposures to the target vegetables that are occurring at home. Comments on the questionnaires provide qualitative feedback on family responses to the recipe and to the program.

Family feedback has helped modify the recipes. For example, families reported that a recipe for ravioli was too complex to prepare for an evening meal by busy families with young children. We removed that recipe from the program. Feedback also provided ideas for improving communication with families. Based on family requests, we now post the recipe of the week in classrooms to inform families at the beginning of each week what will be sent home in the Family Recipe Kit. This helps families arrange to purchase additional ingredients, if necessary, or include the recipe in their meal planning for the week.

At the end of the twenty-four weeks, families participate in focus groups to share the impact of Early Sprouts on their child and family. Focus groups bring together individuals to provide focused feedback on a topic. Focus groups are usually facilitated by someone not directly involved with the program so participants can give honest feedback. Some method of recording the discussion is important. Participants are reassured that their individual comments will not be attributed to them directly.

The Early Sprouts focus group is made up of the families of children who have been in an Early Sprouts classroom. The facilitator is a researcher who does not work directly in classrooms with the curriculum. Our focus group discussions are tape-recorded, with permission of the families, and two staff members listen and take notes. Several meetings are scheduled, and families sign up for the time that is most convenient. Between six and ten participants are ideal, so all can share their ideas. Each session lasts approximately one hour. We use the following four questions to focus the discussion.

1. Describe your family's overall experience with the Early Sprouts program, in particular the Family Recipe Kits. We'll do a "round robin" for the first question to be sure everyone has the chance to talk.

2. As you know, Early Sprouts has focused on providing a seed-to-table experience for children using six target vegetables. To help us gauge the impact of these experiences, please describe any changes you've noticed in your child's eating habits this year, especially their attitudes toward vegetables or their willingness to try new foods.

3. Since you are the experts on your child's involvement, interest, preferences, and style, we need your feedback on how things have gone with Early Sprouts. From your perspective, what worked well in the Early Sprouts program?

4. What suggestions do you have for improving the Early Sprouts program from your family's perspective? Notes on the meeting are transcribed, organized by theme, and reported back to the Early Sprouts program and the focus group participants. This information provides detailed feedback on the impact of the project.

Impact on Children

During the course of the twenty-four week program, we are able to measure a significant increase in children's willingness to taste vegetables. Each child approaches the vegetables, the sensory explorations, and the cooking experiences differently. For example, Keisha tasted all the vegetables the first time they were introduced. Samantha started trying the Early Sprouts snacks around week 12. Logan observed the first half of the entire program and finally licked a vegetable during the last week. Overall, the data show that children become more willing to approach new foods, regardless of how each individual child behaves. One teacher, Elena, sums it up nicely: "Our entire classroom is now more adventurous about tasting new foods."

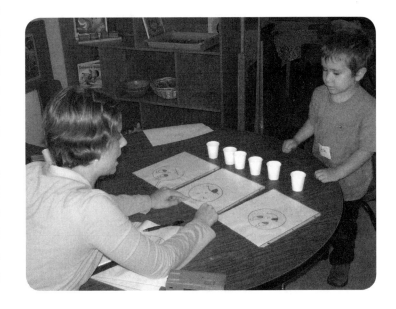

Data show that in general, children's willingness to taste the target and the novel (beets, summer squash, and cauliflower) vegetables increased between week 1 and week 12 of the program. It increased even more between week 13 and the end of the entire 24 weeks. We also observed an increase in children's preference for the target and novel vegetables during the twenty-four weeks. These increases occurred for all vegetables. The increase in children's willingness to taste is most dramatic for the six target vegetables, but it also occurs for the novel vegetables. Children show more willingness to try most vegetables after participating in Early Sprouts. Thus, the results support our hypothesis that Early Sprouts enhances young children's openness to new foods and appears to decrease their innate food neophobia.

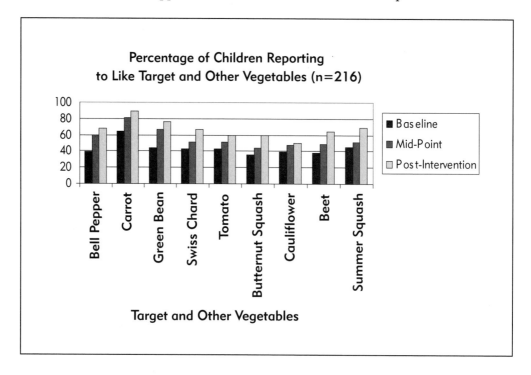

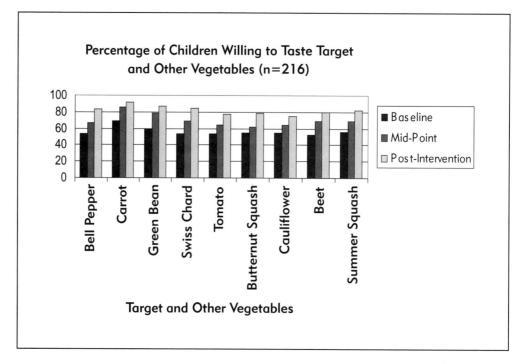

Here are some things children say about Early Sprouts:

"I love greens. Can we cook them again tomorrow?"

"Butternut Squash Pancakes were my favorite. I am going to make these at home."

"I made bell pepper couscous castles for my whole family."

"I had a carrot for breakfast."

"I am leaving early today. Can I pack my ingredients early? I can't go home without my ingredients."

Children's enthusiasm for the Early Sprouts activities also increased. Four-year-old Paul entered the classroom reluctantly one day, wanting to return home with his mother. The teacher commented that lots of exciting activities were going to happen that day. Paul asked, "Are we doing Early Sprouts today? If we are, I'm staying." Families are happy to report that their Early Sprouts child is more open to new foods and less picky than their older children. Although there is a great range of openness to tasting new foods among individual children, we have heard this comment often enough to believe that Early Sprouts is having a positive impact at the dinner table as well as in the classroom.

We see changes in children's willingness to participate. Jackson, a four-year-old, observed the Early Sprouts lessons, participated in sensory explorations and cooking, but refused to taste anything. At the end of the program, during the preference testing, he licked a bell pepper for the first time.

We see the children's interest in gardening expanding as well. Five-year-old Ella reported about her family garden at circle time. "We didn't grow carrots at my house this year. We forgot to plant carrot seeds." Four-year-old José said, "I think we should plant tomatoes, rainbow chard, and squash in our garden. And I will eat them all."

We have learned from families how their child's interest in vegetables has influenced the entire family. Maggie's mother, Andrea, reported that they now have seven different types of squash in the kitchen because of Maggie's insistence that they try new varieties. Maggie loves the produce section of the supermarket and selects something new each week. Children creatively apply the lessons of Early Sprouts to other foods. Anthony's dad, Phil, reported that Anthony tried to convince the family to buy several different types of candy, giggling as he explained, "You're supposed to try new foods!" Children are bringing vegetables in their lunches. Four-year-old Sergei brings chopped Swiss chard in his lunch and tells his friends, "I prefer chard raw."

Impact on Teachers

In our regular meetings with teachers and during training sessions with new staff members, we receive many supportive comments. Teachers are connecting the goals and outcomes of Early Sprouts to their states' early childhood curriculum guidelines and with national curriculum standards sponsored by Head Start and the National Association for the Education of Young Children (NAEYC). Implementing the Early Sprouts curriculum can seem challenging at first, but teachers begin to appreciate the results after they become familiar with the approach. The children really lead the way with their engagement in the curriculum.

When reflecting on the program's impact on her group of pre-K children, Cherie states, "Early Sprouts expands children's ability to observe the world, ask questions, and seek answers. My children approach everything now as scientists. They observe carefully, ask interesting questions, seek out new information, and approach the world with a sense of wonder." Ross, a teacher of three-year-olds, comments, "We have cooked in the classroom before, but never have we been so deliberate and consistent in our approach." Hailey adds, "This program has changed the way our whole classroom approaches new foods. It is really amazing. I always knew it was important to teach our children about nutrition, but I was never really sure how to do that before Early Sprouts."

Teachers have noted the ways that Early Sprouts promotes development and learning in all areas of the curriculum. Jenna, an experienced preschool special educator, says,

> It's more than just nutrition. Some of our children never go to the art table, but they will come over to use the kitchen scissors to cut the chard. Children develop fine-motor coordination when they use the kitchen tools. Their social competence increases as they cooperate on making the recipes. They are learning so much. Each time we return to one of the vegetables, I feel like the children go deeper with their investigation. It's so cool!

Teachers and administrators also note the links to home and family that Early Sprouts supports. Tanya, the director of an employer-sponsored child care center, says it this way:

> We have never done such a good job coordinating what is happening in our classroom with what families are doing at home. The Family Recipe Kits are a perfect way to bridge the classroom and the home environment. It is so exciting to be a part of this initiative. We are really helping our children and their families develop positive attitudes about eating healthy foods.

Impact on Families

Family feedback indicates a range of interest and participation in the project. "I had never eaten chard and now it is a regular in our home. Now we are all looking for new foods in the produce section," declares a father of two children in the program. Families participating in the program represent the full range of dietary habits within our society. Some are vegetarians or cook with whole foods; others use the microwave to reheat take-out meals. But all have become more aware of their food habits because of Early Sprouts. "This program held our family accountable for what we ate and what we had available for snacks—carrots, not chips!" comments one couple. Another mother reports, "Gardening was an important part of this project for my child. This year we planted our first family garden." And families recognize the way the program supports children's food choices: "Early Sprouts works well to expand children's food horizons—it is such a picky stage!"

The families we survey have a range of opinions about the weekly Family Recipe Kits. Some look forward to having something new to cook each week, while others feel they can't keep up. A positive outcome is discovering that children can help with meal preparation, as reflected in this comment: "I had no idea my child could assist with cooking. Now some of our favorite time is spent in the kitchen." Families agree that the Early Sprouts program has a positive impact on their child and on their family. "My whole family is eating better, even my 'I don't eat anything green' husband," states one mother. Another parent says, "I used to battle with my child over eating vegetables. Now my child is requesting specific vegetables at the store and at mealtimes." A common sentiment is expressed by this parent: "Every child and family should have an Early Sprouts experience. My older child is much fussier about food."

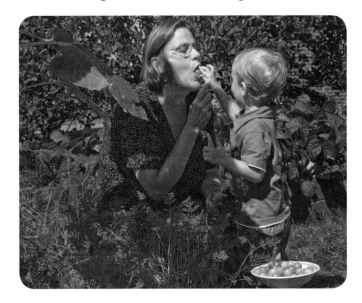

These anecdotes provide substantial, qualitative evidence of positive changes. We see household attitudes toward vegetables changing. We can identify shifts in consumption and purchasing patterns. One preschooler, four-year-old Stefania, began asking to have some of her mother's salad for supper. Now mom and daughter fix salads and eat together. Preschool children are notorious for demanding sweetened cereals and other junk food at the grocery store. Now we hear about the impact of a child's insistence on three colors of bell peppers or two different varieties of squash in the produce section. This "positive pester power" shows us that children's interest in trying new vegetables is influencing entire families.

The following list summarizes the themes gathered from family focus groups:

- Gardening was an important part of the project.
- Children enjoyed the sensory explorations and cooking activities.
- Families got involved in cooking, learning about vegetables, and trying new foods at home.
- Many children liked the raw vegetables, as well as the variety of textures and colors.
- The recipes opened up new ideas for cooking and eating vegetables.
- Sometimes it was hard for families to prepare all of the recipes from the kits.
- Children were sometimes more involved in the process of cooking than in eating the product, and ate more while cooking than at meals.
- Families would like regular information about the project, such as upcoming vegetables and recipes to include at home.
- Early Sprouts works well to expand children's food horizons, especially at an age when they can be picky eaters influenced by social cues, such as advertising, what others are eating, food attitudes of adults, and other external factors.

Conducting research takes time and organization. Tools for formulating data must be implemented with consistency. The resulting data must be analyzed to determine the results of the project. You don't need to include the formal parts of the research to be successful with Early Sprouts. Most likely you will want to gather feedback from teachers, families, and children to gauge the effectiveness of the program in your location. Use the information to make adjustments. Maybe you will want to adjust one of the recipes because it's too simple. Maybe a friend has a great addition to one of the sensory ideas. Maybe one of your families can donate produce, so you substitute their favorite vegetable for one of the ones included here. Our research results should assure you that your investment in this program will yield positive changes in the lives of your children and the adults around them. The rest is up to you.

FOURTEEN

ADAPTING AND ADOPTING
THE EARLY SPROUTS APPROACH

THE EARLY SPROUTS PROGRAM REPRESENTS a commitment to a nutritionally purposeful preschool environment. What does this mean? It means several things. We offer healthy foods in a developmentally appropriate manner. We offer foods for celebrations that follow the Early Sprouts guidelines. We provide multiple opportunities to try a new food. We understand people can begin to like a new food if given time, support, and opportunity to try it. We respect food as something that nourishes us, and we do not use it for other kinds of play. We involve children in gardening, harvesting, and food preparation. We ask adults to model healthy eating behaviors too. We focus on positive food behaviors in children and families. And we involve families in learning experiences. We have found great success with this approach, and we know you will as well.

We recognize that our target vegetables, recipes, and gardening information are directly related to our own location. We encourage you to vary the vegetables to fit your needs. Using our list of vegetables is not necessary. You can substitute spinach or bok choy for Swiss chard, try growing edible pumpkins instead of butternut squash, or replace bell peppers with poblano peppers. Be responsive to your community as you decide on the target vegetables to try. Feel free to adapt and adjust the recipes. And please share your results with us!

Incorporate the Food Philosophy of Early Sprouts

Allow children to serve themselves the amount they think they can eat. Do not force them to finish everything; rather, remind them to take a smaller portion next time. Talk with children about how people develop a liking for new foods over time.

Foods provided for lunch and/or snack should be nutritionally balanced. Follow the principles of reduced fat, sugar, and salt in all the foods you serve. Along with this, work to increase fruit, vegetable, and whole-grain consumption. On days when an Early Sprouts food is not served as snack, provide vegetables or fruit along with a whole-grain cereal or cracker. For birthday celebrations, have children chose between Carrot Muffins and Butternut Squash Muffins for their birthday cake—you can cook either recipe in a cake pan, and children don't always need frosting to make a cake feel special. Holiday parties can also incorporate Early Sprouts recipes. Cherry Tomatoes with Honey Mustard Dip, Carrot Oatmeal Cookies, and Cheddar and Chard Quesadillas are examples of healthy finger foods for classroom parties.

Teaching children to respect food is an important component of the Early Sprouts approach. You can convey your respect for food in a variety of ways. Each sensory activity provides a safe opportunity for children to explore and understand the vegetable. Be purposeful by always concluding the activity with an opportunity to taste the vegetable. This reminds children that the vegetable is a food and not a plaything. Be intentional in the decision to avoid using foods as art materials, craft supplies, or replacement for sand at the sensory table. Work to communicate the difference between exploring food and playing with food. Compost your food scraps whenever possible. Composting serves as a reminder that food can nourish the soil as well as our bodies.

Work to encourage your entire staff to accept and model the same philosophy about food. Teachers and other staff members can demonstrate an adventurous spirit and be willing to taste new foods. Invite adults to sit down and join the children for Early Sprouts snacks and meals. Enthusiastic adults encourage children to try the cooking activities and other vegetable explorations. Children are quick to notice the teacher who consumes a soda during naptime, the one who runs in and out of the classroom to consume morning coffee and a donut, and the one who never eats the Early Sprouts foods. Children are equally quick to notice the teacher who displays enthusiasm for the garden, who eats bell peppers and carrot sticks at lunch, and who eagerly tries each new Early Sprouts recipe. Providing consistency in exposing a child to food can set the stage for a lifetime of healthy eating.

We encourage you to use the Early Sprouts philosophy of offering healthy foods in a developmentally appropriate manner for all of your food-related activities, including family events. At a family event, such as a picnic, encourage families to bring a recipe that includes an Early Sprouts vegetable. Share nutritional guidelines and portion sizes (see chapter 2) with families. This will help them develop healthy lunches or snacks for the classroom. Include information about the recipes and Early Sprouts vegetables in your newsletter. Encourage families to try the recipes at home, and provide tips for involving their children in the cooking process.

Model the Early Sprouts philosophy for families and communicate your approach to food clearly. This is important to the success of the program and the goal of promoting positive eating habits. Through Early Sprouts, we can help families overcome their own fears about new foods. We can remind them of the importance of modeling healthy eating habits for their children. We can teach them that everyone can grow to like a new food. A perfect example is three-year-old Lauren's dad, Dan. Dan picks up Lauren from school each Thursday, which is Early Sprouts Family Recipe Kit day. As soon as Dan enters the room (after greeting Lauren with a hug), he eagerly inquires about the Early Sprouts kit. He asks Lauren about each of the ingredients and humorously investigates the contents of the bag. Typically he concludes this interaction with a comment such as, "Wow, I can't wait to try Sesame Seed Green Beans!" Needless to say, Lauren is a very enthusiastic Early Sprouts participant. Dan reports that the Early Sprouts experience has been a "huge eye-opener" for his family. He and his partner are now much more devoted to creating a healthy food environment for their children. Your program will have successes like Lauren and Dan's when you embrace the Early Sprouts philosophy and approach.

Consider Geography and Cultural Diversity

To date, all of the preschools participating in the Early Sprouts program are located in the Northeast. Our growing season is limited to the five months between the end of May and the middle of October. The Early Sprouts target vegetables will grow in almost any United States Department of Agriculture (USDA) Plant Hardiness Zone. We selected the six vegetables based on their range of colors, shapes, and textures; their varying nutritional profiles; and their ability to grow successfully in the Northeast. However, there are many alternative vegetables from which to choose. For example, we could have easily substituted kale, sweet potatoes, beets, or zucchini. If you live in a geographic area that does not lend itself to easily growing the featured vegetables, select a more suitable group. Try to include something leafy, one root vegetable, and a variety of colors, shapes, and textures. We encourage you to identify vegetables that will work well for your region.

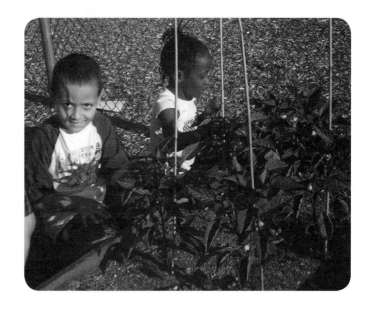

If you are located in an area where you cannot plant a garden, consider container gardening, a porch or rooftop, or set up an indoor vegetable growing lab. Chapter 3 contains information to help you get started in these alternate gardening adventures. Another viable option is to implement the program without a garden.

You can easily use purchased vegetables for the sensory, in-class cooking, and Family Recipe Kit components of the program. Sharing photos of vegetable plants can result in discussions with children about the source of their food. A trip to a nearby farmers' market, farm, backyard garden, grocery store, or neighborhood market can further enhance the experience. Vegetables can be found in many different locations. Be creative with how you help connect the children to the growing process. Remember that one goal is to help children see their connection to the land and the food supply.

The Early Sprouts program can be used as a way to celebrate and explore ethnic and cultural diversity in your classroom. As you'll recall from chapters 8–11, several Early Sprouts recipes are drawn from differing cultural backgrounds, such as wontons, quesadillas, and homemade pizza. Perhaps you can select a few vegetables from ethnic cuisines as part of your Early Sprouts program. Bok choy (Chinese), edamame (Japanese), chili peppers (Central and South American), and eggplant (Greek) can all be grown in your garden. Offering a range of recipes supports all children and their families in developing an understanding of diversity.

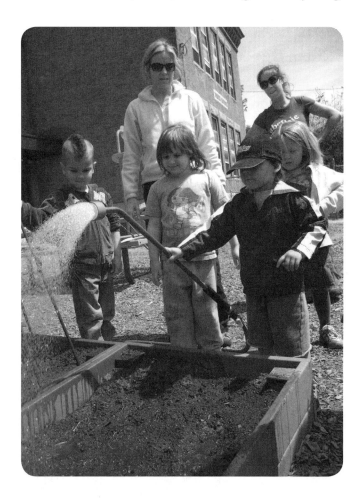

Zhen, a four-year-old boy from China, was a participant in the Early Sprouts program. Zhen's family owns and operates a restaurant. One day, Zhen noticed the wonton wrappers coming out of the classroom refrigerator. For the first time, he decided to participate in the Early Sprouts cooking project. While the other participating children and adults fumbled through their wonton production, Zhen was quick to demonstrate a far more efficient way. This experience provided a perfect opportunity to talk about Chinese culture. It also provided Zhen with an opportunity to share his cultural knowledge. And it showed his family that their cultural background was valued by his preschool.

Your use of specific vegetables in the Early Sprouts program can be flexible. The approach used to introduce and reinforce a new food should be consistent. Provide the children with multiple opportunities to explore, taste, and cook each individual vegetable in a supportive social setting. Remember: it can take five to ten exposures for young children to become familiar with a new food.

Gather Support for Your Program

Many local businesses will be excited about your school's garden project. Local hardware stores, lumberyards, and building supply companies may be willing to donate or substantially discount the material needed to build and maintain your garden beds. Chain and local grocery stores, natural food stores, or food co-ops may be willing support your program through food donations or discounts. Garden supply stores may be able to provide seeds, seedlings, and garden equipment. Finally, monetary support can be sought from local charitable organizations.

Many hands make for light work in the garden. We suggest seeking out volunteers to assist in building and maintaining your gardens. Local Habitat for Humanity chapters may be excited to provide a garden construction team to assist in making the raised beds. Master gardeners, cooperative extension office staff, garden clubs, service clubs, farmers, parents, and restaurant owners may be willing to devote some of their time to help ensure the success of your program.

Consider carefully how the Early Sprouts program can best work for you, your classroom, and/or your center. Perhaps you want to implement the entire program as outlined in this book. Perhaps you want to begin with certain components. For example, in the first year, you may want to focus on the classroom activities. Maybe you decide to feature one vegetable instead of all six. Whether you decide to start with one tomato plant growing in a large pot or choose to build a huge play yard garden, your decision will be a positive step for you and your preschoolers. You will be helping create a preschool experience that fosters the development of lifelong healthy eating habits. And it may even be so much fun that you'll naturally want to expand your program!

Ellen Edge, preschool director, sums it up this way:

Since Early Sprouts began, we have observed a marked change in our children's attitudes about foods. We have seen a rise in consumption of vegetables, as well as an increased appreciation for produce and a greater willingness to try new foods. Our relationships with our families are stronger and more collaborative. Our outdoor play environment has been enhanced by the gardens, and Early Sprouts has led to innovative and emerging curricula across multiple learning domains. Early Sprouts has enhanced our programming in ways that go beyond nutrition.

FIFTEEN

PARTING WORDS

Dr. Susan Lynch, pediatrician and pediatric lipids specialist, is committed to solving the problem of childhood obesity and encouraging healthy eating habits and regular exercise for New Hampshire's children. Her words aptly summarize the goal of the Early Sprouts program: "It's easier to teach a behavior than to change one." Our primary focus is on instilling positive dietary habits in young children. Working with preschool children provides an ideal opportunity to teach healthy behaviors around food and nutrition. In recognition of the many different factors that influence children's dietary habits, we have taken a comprehensive approach and drawn on many fields of knowledge.

We began with our knowledge of child development. Preschool children are developmentally ready to learn, solve problems, and participate in many activities of daily living. Because young children are managing their eating, sleeping, dressing, and toileting, they respond well to being given responsibility in these areas. We have incorporated these developmental characteristics into planning sensory explorations and cooking activities. As you have seen, we have also drawn from research on the formation of food preferences and the number of exposures needed for children to become familiar with a food.

The Early Sprouts approach is based on knowledge gained from theories of behavioral change. These psychological theories posit ways that human beings learn and adapt; they suggest strategies to support learning new behaviors or changing existing ones. They guide us in supporting children's self-efficacy through multiple small, yet progressive, steps. Children's skills and knowledge about foods, cooking, and gardening increase. Recurring opportunities to taste, explore, and cook with specific vegetables result in repeated positive feedback from adults and peers. These experiences contribute to the expansion of healthy eating behaviors.

Other developmental models identify multiple layers of influence on individuals, including those of the family, school, community, and culture. These models add another source of support for the Early Sprouts approach. We have created purposeful interventions at several levels: individual, school, family. We have drawn connections between families and their community. We have introduced the culture of food production to all involved through the implementation of a play yard garden and the seed-to-table approach.

Early Sprouts helps children overcome their innate fear of new foods by providing multiple opportunities to explore and taste vegetables. The program helps children gain an understanding of where their food comes from. It also creates an environment that supports healthy eating through in-class cooking and sensory explorations and garden-based activities in the play yard. Early Sprouts interacts with children's home environments by bringing critical components of the experience into their homes and directly involving families through take-home Family Recipe Kits and family events. We know that Early Sprouts has positively influenced the preschool food environment. Centers have changed their snack menus to include more fruits, vegetables, whole grains, and low-fat dairy products. Traditional birthday cakes have been replaced with healthy carrot and butternut squash baked goods. Families are sending more vegetables in children's lunches and communicating their enthusiasm for the changes.

The Early Sprouts program has many components. Each is grounded in a deep understanding of young children. Each comes from our knowledge of research and theory and from our experience putting this knowledge into practice. Each plays an important role in the overall program. We are pleased that you are considering joining us in the Early Sprouts approach. Your effort will be a step toward supporting young children in the development of healthy eating habits. Collectively, we can help reverse America's childhood obesity epidemic and create lifelong health for young children.

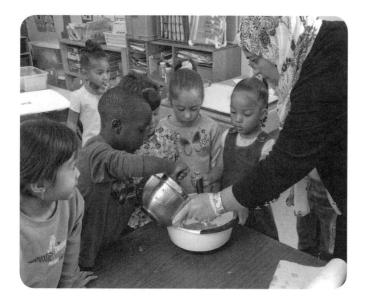

⌐∾ **APPENDIX A** ∾⌐

VITAMINS AND SELECTED
MINERALS CHART

VITAMINS	MAJOR ROLES	SUGGESTED SOURCES
Vitamin A	Helps maintain skin, mucous membranes, bones, teeth, and hair. Plays a key role in vision.	Dark leafy greens (chard, kale, collards), winter squash (butternut), red bell peppers, carrots, sweet potatoes, and broccoli.
Vitamin D	Helps the body absorb calcium and supports bone growth and development.	Low-fat dairy, salmon, and fortified cereals.
Vitamin E	Helps form red blood cells and serves as an antioxidant.	Seeds, nuts, whole grains, plant oils, avocado, and dark leafy greens.
Vitamin K	Important for blood clotting and bone health.	Dark leafy greens, broccoli, green beans, and cabbage.
Thiamin (Vitamin B_1)	Critical for nervous system function. Enables the use of carbohydrates for energy.	Whole grains, wheat germ/bran, nuts, seeds, orange juice, and beans.
Riboflavin (Vitamin B_2)	Enables the use of foods for energy. Essential for healthy skin, hair, nails, and eyes.	Whole grains, dark leafy greens, fortified cereals, broccoli, low-fat dairy, and raw mushrooms.
Niacin (Vitamin B_3)	Assists with digestive and nervous system functioning and essential for metabolizing protein and carbohydrates.	Mushrooms, wheat bran, tuna, chicken, turkey, asparagus, and peanuts.
Pyridoxine (Vitamin B_6)	Has a key role in metabolism and helps red blood cells form. Important for healthy pregnancies.	Bananas, avocado, whole wheat bread, cantaloupe, pecans, acorn squash, salmon, and blackstrap molasses.
Cobalamin (Vitamin B_{12})	Helps red blood cells form. Prevents anemia and promotes growth in children.	Fortified breakfast cereals, yogurt, milk, eggs, and meat.
Folic acid	Critical for the formation of red blood cells, assists in healing, aids in metabolism of proteins, and contributes to normal growth.	Dark leafy greens, broccoli, fortified breakfast cereals, whole and fortified grains, lima beans, and sunflower seeds.
Pantothenic acid	Affects all vital body functions. Helps ward off infections and speeds recovery from illness.	Whole grains, green vegetables, fortified cereals, and peanuts.

Biotin	Assists in metabolizing proteins and fats and prevents hair loss.	Nuts, eggs, and low-fat dairy.
Vitamin C	Critical for healthy teeth, gums, and bones. Essential for proper functioning of thyroid glands.	Tomatoes, bell peppers, strawberries, cabbage, cantaloupe, sweet potato, apples, citrus fruits, and strawberries.

SELECTED MINERALS	MAJOR ROLES	SUGGESTED SOURCES
Calcium	Necessary for bone and tooth formation, heart function, blood clotting, and muscle contraction.	Dark leafy greens, dairy products (low-fat milk and yogurt), oats, navy beans, almonds, millet, broccoli, and sunflower seeds.
Phosphorus	Works with calcium and helps build bones and teeth.	Low-fat cheese, yogurt, milk, beans, lentils, tofu, fortified cereals, lean beef, and peanut butter.
Magnesium	Assists with muscle development, healthy bones and heart.	Nuts, seeds, dark leafy greens, beans, tomatoes, and brown rice.
Potassium	Critical for muscle contraction and normal heart functioning.	Tomato, apricots, kidney beans, yogurt, lima beans, whole grains, bananas, and zucchini.
Sodium	Regulates fluid and acid-base balance.	Celery, romaine lettuce, watermelon, and sea salt.
Iron	Assists with the formation of hemoglobin, which carries oxygen in the blood. Helps resists stress and disease.	Lean beef, dark leafy greens, lentils, oat bran, and dry beans.
Zinc	Component in enzymes and insulin that aids in wound healing, growth, tissue repair, and sexual development.	Brown rice, yogurt, pumpkin seeds, oatmeal, lentils, whole-wheat/rye bread, and beans.
Selenium	Strengthens immune system and serves as antioxidant.	Brazil nuts, nuts, whole grains, brown rice, lean beef, oatmeal, and chicken.

⌒ APPENDIX B ⌒

PREPARING THE GARDEN SITE

This section will help guide you through constructing your garden's raised beds, provide information about soil and soil preparation, and offer tips on planning and planting your garden.

Constructing Garden Beds

When you have the size, shape, and design of your garden created, you're ready to select building materials. Before building our first garden beds, we spent a lot of time researching the characteristics and comparing the costs of various building materials. We concluded that using composite decking for the primary material of the raised bed boxes was the best choice. Composite decking, which is sold under various brand names, is a nontoxic, chemical-free combination of wood and plastic. The plastic protects the wood from insect and weather damage; the wood protects the plastic from damaging UV rays. Millions of pounds of recycled and reclaimed plastics and wood are converted into this rot-free, long-lasting material. The raw materials used to make this decking come from recycled plastic grocery bags, reclaimed pallet wrap, and hardwood sawdust. Composite decking is free from cracks and splinters and never requires painting or sanding. These characteristics combine to make it ideal for raised-bed children's gardens.

Some lumberyards may suggest pressure-treated wood as a less expensive alternative. Pressure-treated wood is injected with chemicals that kill termites and preserve the wood. Be careful when considering this alternative, because pressure-treated woods contain harmful chemicals, such as creosote, pentachlorophenol, and other toxic chemicals that may leach into your soil and vegetables. Even manufacturers of this type of wood recommend that adults use gloves when handling it and wear breathing masks when in contact with sawdust from the wood. Manufacturers also recommend that young children be kept from contact with the product. Splinters from pressure-treated wood cause serious infections because of the chemicals used to treat the wood. Health and safety guidelines often prohibit the use of pressure-treated wood for children's play yard equipment or require regular surface treatment to protect consumers from contact with the chemicals in it.

Even though composite decking is initially more expensive than wood, we believe it is the better choice because of its durability, safety, and more positive environmental impact.

You will need corner posts for your raised beds. We recommend composite decking or cedar or redwood posts (also rot resistant) to serve as the corners of your raised beds. These can be installed without staining or painting. Finally, before leaving the lumberyard, be sure to purchase a large box of decking screws. Standard screws will easily become stripped in this strong and durable material.

When building your raised beds, leave the bottoms of the boxes open for soil drainage. It is important that a water-permeable layer be placed at the bottom of the box. This layer allows water to exit and assists in keeping soil in. We recommend using landscape cloth for this purpose. Here are the directions for building the frames for your raised beds:

1. Using 4-inch by 4-inch by 8-foot cedar posts, cut four 10-inch lengths for each bed. This will provide the maximum number of pieces, leaving the least amount of waste.

2. Cut the composite decking into the desired lengths. Assemble the two longest sides of the box first on a firm, flat surface. Lay two of the cedar posts down, set two of the 1-inch by 6-inch pieces of composite decking on top, and align the edges of the decking with the edges of the cedar posts. Align the edges of the decking with the bottom edge of the post. Reserve extra posts for additional support, as described in step 7.

3. Fasten the decking to the posts with composite decking screws (see Garden Construction Graphic A on the next page). Using the composite decking screws is important because they are self-drilling and will prevent "puckering" of the composite decking.

4. Stand the two assembled sides up on the narrow top edge, making sure they are approximately parallel. Space them so they are the same distance apart as the short pieces you will be attaching in the next step. The 4-inch by 4-inch posts will allow the two sides to stand. Remember that the bottom edges of the posts and decking should be flush.

5. Set one piece from the short side of the bed in place, and fasten it to the corner post. Fasten the second piece on the same end (see Garden Construction Graphic B on the next page).

6. Fasten the two pieces on the opposite end as you did in step 5.

7. It may be necessary to provide bracing at the midpoint of boxes longer than 6 feet to prevent them from bowing once they are filled with soil.

This can be done either by adding 4-inch by 4-inch post to both sides, fastening them as you would a corner post, or by using scrap decking material attached with shorter screws. After the braces are fastened, connect them with a cross member to provide support (see Garden Construction Graphic A for details).

GARDEN CONSTRUCTION GRAPHIC A

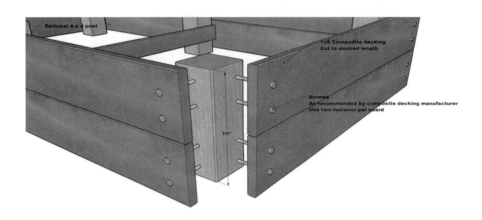

GARDEN CONSTRUCTION GRAPHIC B

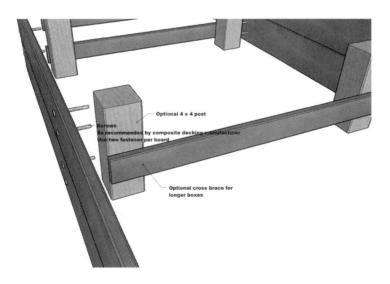

Soil and Soil Preparation

The ideal garden soil is fertile, deep, loose, well drained, rich in organic matter, and free of weeds and disease organisms. If your soil does not meet this definition, you can transform your less-than-ideal soil with a little preparation and work.

Because garden soil needs appropriate nutrients and an appropriate acid-to-base (pH) balance for plants to grow well, you should have your soil tested before you begin planting. Soil testing reveals the nature and quality of your garden soil and suggests what you should add to balance ingredients for growing plants. Your local USDA Cooperative Extension Service has information on soil testing and can often complete the test for about $20. Submit your soil samples well in advance of planting time if possible, and repeat soil testing each year. The report specifies your soil's pH level, indicates any need for phosphorus, potassium, lime, and various trace elements, and makes recommendations to bring your soil into balance. Be sure to select elemental organic fertilizers to amend your soil. Bone meal, greensand, and rock phosphate are derived from natural sources and are well suited to redressing soil imbalances.

In a well-drained soil, water moves quickly and never compromises air movement. Without good drainage, roots are denied oxygen and struggle to develop and function properly. A soil that contains too much clay dries too slowly. A soil with too much sand dries too quickly. Clay and sandy soils can be greatly improved by adding organic matter. Manure, composted leaves, sawdust, bark, and peat moss can improve the quality of your soil.

You will want to further enrich your soil by adding organic matter to enhance water retention and good drainage. Use both animal- and plant-derived compost, and select processed, composted animal manure products (in bags) to minimize risk. For green compost, use leaves and plant-based kitchen waste, such as fruit, vegetable, coffee grinds, tea leaves, and eggshells. Before each growing season, add an additional 1- to 2-inch layer of compost or composted manure, and work it into the soil before planting (see the Composting section, page 195, to learn more about making your own compost).

After the garden bed is filled with soil and enriched with the organic matter and soil amendments indicated by your soil tests, you will want to let the soil settle before you plant. Adding earthworms, if they are not present in your native soil, is a must. Earthworms aerate the soil and add nutrients in their waste products. Garden soil naturally compacts over time, especially when people walk on the surface. Soil preparation is an annual task that is part of the excitement of preparing to plant the garden. Prior to planting your garden each year, you should till the soil, either with a mechanical tiller or by hand-turning the top 6 to 10 inches of soil with a garden fork or spade. This loosens and aerates the soil, allowing seedlings' tiny roots to expand into the soil and soak up water and nutrients.

Planning and Planting the Garden

Start by sketching a diagram of your garden bed. Give thought to the direction the sun travels in relationship to your garden beds, and notice when certain areas are shaded. Some plants need more direct sunlight; others might do well with partial shade or fewer hours of direct sun. Consider the predicted height of each garden plant. Ideally, shorter vegetable plants should not be shaded by taller ones. Plant the taller plants in the northern part of the garden to minimize their impact on sunlight for the shorter plants. To determine how many seedlings to buy or seeds to sow, consider your total growing space and how much space is needed between plants. Following the guidelines on your seed packages or seedling tag, calculate how many plants will fit into each row. Seed catalogues also have great information on spacing seeds or seedlings.

Next, based on the USDA Plant Hardiness Zone for your region, determine if you will plant your garden with seedlings, seeds, or a combination of both. In New Hampshire, for example, we can start butternut squash, carrots, Swiss chard, and green beans by sowing the seeds directly in the garden. Tomato and bell pepper plants, however, need to be planted in the garden as seedlings because of our short growing season.

Organic seeds can be purchased from most gardening supply stores or online. For a list of sources, see appendix C, Recommended Organic Seed Sources, page 197. Many gardening supply stores, greenhouses, and farmers' markets sell seedlings. A local organic farmer may be willing to contract with you to start your seeds indoors. Check out www.localharvest.org to find a local farmer or farmers' market.

Composting

By composting organic kitchen scraps, yard waste, and other plant matter, you can harness microbes, worms, and insects to decompose materials under controlled conditions and turn them into rich, luscious soil. Bacteria, fungi, worms, and insects each play a role in creating compost from food scraps and dead plants. A play yard composting system uses food scraps that would otherwise be thrown away to create nutrient-rich compost and helps your garden be self-sustaining. As a bonus, a compost pile contributes to your garden's role in teaching children about the cycle of life.

The ingredients for making successful compost include air, water, plant-based organic materials, various microbes, insects, and worms, and enough time for decomposition to occur. Fruit and vegetable scraps, eggshells, coffee grounds, and tea leaves make ideal composting materials and are considered *green matter*, meaning they are nitrogen rich. Play yard leaves, straw, dead flowers, even shredded newspaper are carbon rich and called *brown matter*. Your compost pile needs layers of brown matter alternating with layers of the green matter you collect from Early Sprouts activities.

Both types of compost materials are important to the composting process; an ideal mixture contains a ratio of three parts of brown to one part of green matter.

Note: Meat scraps, dairy products, fatty trash, and household pet or human waste should *never* be added to the compost pile. These materials attract animal pests, create odors, and do not break down effectively. Likewise, nonbiodegradable items, such as plastic containers, do not belong in the compost pile. You may want to avoid putting weeds or clippings that have gone to seed into the compost bin you will use to nourish your garden because unless the compost heats up to very high temperatures, the seeds will survive and are likely to sprout in your garden when you use the compost the next year.

It is important to keep the compost pile moist, but not soggy, and to provide air circulation. Every few weeks, use a garden fork to turn the pile. To simplify turning the pile, select a compost container that tumbles. Many garden supply stores sell enclosed composting containers starting at about $100 that are ideal for play yards because they do not attract unwanted creatures. Landfills and other waste disposal centers often have these containers available, especially in communities that emphasize recycling and reducing the waste stream. Compost activators can speed up the process of composting but are usually unnecessary if you are patient. Gardening books, garden supply businesses, farmers, cooperative extension staff, and the Internet offer good sources of information about composting.

Recommended Organic Seed Sources

Fedco Co-operative Seeds
PO Box 520
Waterville Valley, ME 04903-0520
Phone: 207-873-7333
www.fedcoseeds.com

High Mowing Organic Seeds
76 Quarry Road
Wolcott, VT 05680
Phone: 802-472-6174
www.highmowingseeds.com

Johnny's Selected Seeds
955 Benton Avenue
Winslow, ME 04901-2601
Phone: 877-564-6697
www.johnnyseeds.com

Seeds of Change
PO Box 15700
Santa Fe, NM 87507-5700
Phone: 888-762-7333
www.seedsofchange.com

Seed Savers Exchange
3094 North Winn Road
Decorah, IA 52101
Phone: 563-382-5990
www.seedsavers.org

GARDENING AND VEGETABLE RESOURCES

BOOKS AND ARTICLES

Cotner, S. Vegetable gardening in containers. Aggie Horticulture Network. College Station, Tex.: The Agriculture Program of the Texas A&M University System. http://aggiehorticulture.tamu.edu/extension/container/container.html

Ebeling, E., ed. 2003. *Basic composting: all the skills and tools you need to get started.* Mechanicsburg, PA: Stackpole Books.

Gussow, J. D. 2001. *This organic life: Confessions of a suburban homesteader.* White River Junction, VT: Chelsea Green.

Jeavons, J. 2006. *How to grow more vegetables (and fruits, nuts, berries, grains, and other crops) than you ever thought possible on less land than you can imagine.* 7th ed. Berkeley: Ten Speed Press.

Kruger, A., ed. 2005. *Rodale's illustrated encyclopedia of organic gardening.* New York: DK Publishing.

National Gardening Association (NGA) offers a Web site focused on gardening with children, which can be found at www.kidsgardening.com. 1100 Dorset Street, South Burlington, VT 05403. http://www.kidsgardening.org.

Stoecklin, V. Developmentally appropriate gardening for young children. http://www.whitehutchinson.com/children/articles/gardening.shtml

WEB RESOURCES

American Dietetic Association
http://www.eatright.org

Head Start Regulations
http://eclkc.ohs.acf.hhs.gov/hslc

Local Harvest
http://www.localharvest.org

My Dad's Vegetable Garden [Dept. Biology, James Madison University]
http://www.jmu.edu/biology/k12/garden.parts.htm

NAEYC (National Association for the Education of Young Children) Early
Childhood Program Standards
http://www.naeyc.org/academy/standards

Vegetables
- Bell peppers
  http://www.urbanext.uiuc.edu/veggies/peppers1.html
- Butternut squash
  http://www.extension.iastate.edu
- Carrots
  http://www.carrotmuseum.co.uk
  http://www.farmdirectcoop.org
- Green beans
  http://www.greenbeansnmore.com/index.htm
- Swiss chard
  http://www.whfoods.com/foodstoc.php
  http://www.cliffordawright.com
  http://www.justhungry.com
- Tomatoes
  http://www.growtomatoes.com

USDA (United States Department of Agriculture)
- Food Pyramid
  http://www.mypyramid.gov
- Plant Hardiness Zones
  http://www.usna.usda.gov/hardzone

BOOKS ABOUT COOKING
WITH AND FOR CHILDREN

Beach, M., and J. Kauffman. 2006. *Simply in season children's cookbook.* Scottdale, PA: Herald Press.

Colker, L. 2005. *The cooking book: Fostering young children's learning and delight.* Washington, DC: National Association for the Education of Young Children.

Cooper, A., and L. Holmes. 2006. *Lunch lessons: Changing the way we feed our children.* New York: Collins.

Katzen, M. 2005. *Salad people and more real recipes: A new cookbook for preschoolers & up.* Berkeley, CA: Tricycle Press.

Katzen, M., and A. Henderson. 1994. *Pretend soup and other real recipes: A cookbook for preschoolers & up.* Berkeley, CA: Tricycle Press.

Nestle, M. 2006. *What to eat: An aisle-by-aisle guide to savvy food choices and good eating.* New York: North Point Press.

Schlosser, E., and C. Wilson. 2006. *Chew on this: Everything you didn't want to know about fast food.* Boston: Houghton Mifflin.

Waters, A. 1992. *Fanny at Chez Panisse: A child's restaurant adventures with 46 recipes.* New York: William Morrow.

﹂ ABOUT THE AUTHORS ﹃

Karrie Kalich, PhD, RD, LD (kkalich@keene.edu), is associate professor in the Department of Health Science, Nutrition at Keene State College. Dr. Kalich is the creator of Early Sprouts. She has spent more than fourteen years in childhood obesity prevention research. She earned her doctoral degree in Nutrition, Science and Policy from Tufts University. Dr. Kalich consults on health and nutrition topics around the region and has been recognized for her work with Early Sprouts by many colleagues around the country and by the acting U.S. Surgeon General, who presented Dr. Kalich with the Surgeons General's Champion Award, which is given to individuals for "implementing programs to help kids stay active, encourage kids' healthy eating habits, and promote healthy choices."

Dottie Bauer, EdD (dbauer@keene.edu), is professor of Early Childhood Education in the Department of Education at Keene State College. A former preschool teacher, Dr. Bauer earned her doctoral degree from the University of Massachusetts Amherst and specializes in early childhood curriculum development and teacher preparation. Dr. Bauer has been active in state and national accrediting body activities.

Deirdre McPartlin, MEd (dmcpartl@keene.edu), academic program coordinator for the Child Development Center at Keene State College, is responsible for teaching methods in early childhood education. She received her master's degree in Foundations of Education from Antioch New England Graduate School. Ms. McPartlin has extensive experience in early childhood supervision, including curriculum development for young children.

Please share your experiences and suggestions with us. We welcome your new ideas and suggestions for improving the explorations and recipes we have developed. We are eager to learn about your Early Sprouts experience.

~ REFERENCES ~

American Dietetic Association. Food and nutrition information. http://www
.eatright.org (accessed March 3, 2008).

Bellows, L., and J. Anderson. 2006. The food friends: Encouraging preschoolers to
try new foods. *Young Children* 61(3): 37–39.

Birch, L. L. 1979. Preschool children's food preferences and consumption patterns.
Journal of Nutrition Education 11(4): 189–92.

Birch, L. L., and J. A. Fisher. 1996. Experience and children's eating behaviors.
In *Why we eat what we eat: the psychology of eating*, ed. E. D. Capaldi, 113–41.
Washington, DC: American Psychological Association.

———. 1995. Appetite and eating behavior in children. *Pediatric Clinics of North
America* 42: 931–53.

Birch, L. L., and D. W. Marlin. 1982. I don't like it; I never tried it: Effects of
exposure to food on two-year-old children's food preferences. *Appetite* 4: 353–60.

Birch, L. L., S. I. Zimmerman, and H. Hind. 1980. The influence of social-affec-
tive context on the formation of children's food preferences. *Child Development*
51: 856–61.

Bredekamp, S., and C. Copple, eds. 1997. *Developmentally appropriate practice in
early childhood programs.* Rev. ed. Washington, DC: National Association for the
Education of Young Children.

Cadwell, L. B. 1997. *Bringing Reggio Emilia home: An innovative approach to early
childhood education.* New York: Teachers College Press.

Carson, R. 1965. *The sense of wonder.* New York: Harper & Row.

Copley, J. V. 2000. *The young child and mathematics.* Washington, DC: National Association for the Education of Young Children.

Curtis, D., and M. Carter. 2003. *Designs for living and learning: Transforming early childhood environments.* St. Paul, MN: Redleaf Press.

Enns, C. W., S. J. Mickle, and J. D. Goldman. 2002. Trends in food and nutrient intake by children in the United States. *Family Economics and Nutrition Review* 14(2): 56–69.

Fleischman, P. 2004. *Seedfolks.* New York: HarperCollins.

Forest, H. 1998. *Stone soup.* Little Rock, AR: August House.

Galinsky, E. 1987. *The six stages of parenthood.* Reading, MA: Addison-Wesley.

Gallo, A.E. 1999. Food advertising in the United States. Chapter 9 in *America's eating habits: changes and consequences*, ed. Elizabeth Frazao. Washington, DC: U.S. Department of Agriculture, Economic Research Service, Food and Rural Economics Division. Agriculture Information Bulletin No. 750. 173–180.

Harms, T., R. M. Clifford, and D. Cryer. 2005. *Early childhood environment rating scale.* Rev. ed. New York: Teachers College Press.

Isbell, R., and B. Exelby. 2001. *Early environments that work.* Beltsville, MD: Gryphon House.

Johnson, S. L., and L. L. Birch. 1994. Parents' and children's adiposity and eating style. *Pediatrics* 94(5): 653–61.

Jones, E., and J. Nimmo. 1994. *Emergent curriculum.* Washington, DC: National Association for the Education of Young Children.

Katz, L. G., and S. C. Chard. 2000. *Engaging children's minds: The project approach.* Stamford, CT: Ablex Publishing.

Krauss, R. 1945. *The carrot seed.* New York: Harper and Row.

Louv, R. 2005. *Last child in the woods: Saving our children from nature-deficit disorder.* Chapel Hill: Algonquin Books.

Marotz, L. R. 2009. *Health, safety, and nutrition for the young child*, 7th ed. Clifton Park, NY: Delmar Learning.

Mooney, C. G. 2000. *Theories of childhood: An introduction to Dewey, Montessori, Erikson, Piaget, and Vygotsky.* St. Paul, MN: Redleaf Press.

Morris, J., and S. Zidenberg-Cherr. 2002. Garden-enhanced nutrition curriculum improves fourth-grade schoolchildren's knowledge of nutrition and preferences for some vegetables. *Journal of the American Dietetic Association* 102(1): 91–93.

Muñoz, K. A., S. M. Krebs-Smith, R. Ballard-Barbash, and L. E. Cleveland. 1997. Food intakes of U. S. children and adolescents compared with recommendations. *Pediatrics* 100 (3): 323–29.

NAEYC. 2007. *NAEYC Early childhood program standards and accreditation criteria: The mark of quality in early childhood education.* Rev. ed. Washington, DC: National Association for the Education of Young Children.

Nanney, M. S., S. Johnson, M. Elliott, and D. Haire-Joshu. 2007. Frequency of eating homegrown produce is associated with higher intake among parents and their preschool-aged children in rural Missouri. *Journal of the American Dietetic Association* 107(4): 577–84.

National Gardening Association. USDA hardiness zone finder. http://www.garden .org. (accessed March 3, 2008)

Nimmo, J., and B. Hallett. 2008. Childhood in the garden: A place to encounter natural and social diversity. *Young Children* 63(1): 32–38. http://www.journal. naeyc.org/btj/200801.

Penn State Live. 2005. New research center to tackle childhood obesity epidemic. September 1. http://live.psu.edu/story/13259.

Produce Oasis. Is the tomato a fruit or vegetable? http://www.produceoasis.com/. (accessed March 14, 2008)

Rudney, G. L. 2005. *Every teacher's guide to working with parents.* Thousand Oaks, CA: Corwin Press.

Satter, E. 2000. *Child of mine: Feeding with love and good sense.* Boulder, CO: Bull Publishing.

Sullivan, S. A., and L. L. Birch. 1994. Infant dietary experience and acceptance of solid foods. *Pediatrics* 93(2): 271–77.

United States Department of Agriculture. USDA Food Guide Pyramid. http://mypyramid.gov/. (accessed March 3, 2008)

U. S. Department of Health and Human Services and U. S. Department of Agriculture. 2005. *Dietary guidelines for Americans.* Washington, DC: USDA.

Wardlaw, G., and J. Hampl. 2007. *Perspectives in nutrition.* Boston: McGraw-Hill Higher Education.

Witt, S. D., and H. A. Spencer. 2004. Using educational interventions to improve the hand washing habits of preschool children. *Early Childhood Development and Care* 174(5): 461-71.